HEALTH ISSUES IN CHINESE CONTEXTS

NURSING RESEARCH

A CHINESE PERSPECTIVE

ZENOBIA C.Y. CHAN
EDITOR

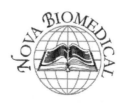

Nova Biomedical Books
New York

For permission to use material from this book please contact us:
Telephone 631-231-7269; Fax 631-231-8175
Web Site: http://www.novapublishers.com

NOTICE TO THE READER

The Publisher has taken reasonable care in the preparation of this book, but makes no expressed or implied warranty of any kind and assumes no responsibility for any errors or omissions. No liability is assumed for incidental or consequential damages in connection with or arising out of information contained in this book. The Publisher shall not be liable for any special, consequential, or exemplary damages resulting, in whole or in part, from the readers' use of, or reliance upon, this material. Any parts of this book based on government reports are so indicated and copyright is claimed for those parts to the extent applicable to compilations of such works.

Independent verification should be sought for any data, advice or recommendations contained in this book. In addition, no responsibility is assumed by the publisher for any injury and/or damage to persons or property arising from any methods, products, instructions, ideas or otherwise contained in this publication.

This publication is designed to provide accurate and authoritative information with regard to the subject matter covered herein. It is sold with the clear understanding that the Publisher is not engaged in rendering legal or any other professional services. If legal or any other expert assistance is required, the services of a competent person should be sought. FROM A DECLARATION OF PARTICIPANTS JOINTLY ADOPTED BY A COMMITTEE OF THE AMERICAN BAR ASSOCIATION AND A COMMITTEE OF PUBLISHERS.

Additional color graphics may be available in the e-book version of this book.

Library of Congress Cataloging-in-Publication Data

Chan, Zenobia C. Y.
  Nursing research : a Chinese perspective / Zenobia C. Y. Chan.
    p. ; cm.
  Includes bibliographical references and index.
  ISBN 978-1-61209-833-3 (hardcover)
  1. Nursing--Research--Methodology. 2. Nursing--Research--China. I. Title.
  [DNLM: 1. Nursing Research--methods. WY 20.5]
  RT81.5.C434 2011
  610.73072'051--dc22
                        2011005834

Published by Nova Science Publishers, Inc. † New York

Contents

Preface

Nursing research plays an important role in the development of nursing care. Nursing care has developed into an evidence-based practice and research studies could provide more evidence in this practice, thereby enabling the authors to evaluate the effectiveness of the care provided. Research should help create a scientific knowledge baseline for nursing practice which would include health promotion, protection and prevention from illness, optimization of health conditions for not only the people who are critically ill, but also for those who are healthy. This new book presents and discusses nursing research, as well as how through research a cost-effective health care system can be developed.

Chapter 1- There is no doubt that nursing research plays an important role on the development of nursing care. Nursing care have been developed into evidence-based practice and research studies is therefore a must, which will provide more evidence in nursing practice and thus can evaluate the effectiveness of nursing care provided. Understanding the history of the nursing research could help the authors to realize the development of the nursing research and its relationship with other aspects of nursing such as the development of nursing education and change in nursing role. Research will help to build up a scientific knowledge-base for nursing practice which includes health promotion, protection and prevention from illness, optimization of health condition for not only the people who are critically ill, but also for those who are healthy thus, providing holistic care to everyone. Through research, a cost-effective health care system can be developed and also provide an ensuring standard of nursing care.

Chapter 2- This essay provides a brief review of positivist paradigm. The aim of this paper gives a basic understanding of positivist paradigm, the characteristics and its influences to nursing research. Positivist paradigm is commonly used in research that acquires knowledge from observing the fact in the natural world objectively with scientific measurement. And iIt is dominant and has great influences to nursing research development. In this essay, the historical and philosophical aspects will be first overviewed first. Next, the ontology, epistemology and methodology in philosophical aspects will be described briefly, and the characteristics of the paradigm are followed. Finally, the relationship between positivist paradigm and nursing research development will be discussed as the conclusion.

Chapter 3- This article demonstrates the positivistic paradigm in nursing discipline. The importance of positivism and paradigm is briefly described. The philosophical assumptions of positivistic paradigm in ontology, epistemology, axiology, rhetorical structure, and methodology are discussed for having a better understanding. A quantitative research example was used for the illustration of assumptions. The Aapplication on positivistic paradigm in research is quantitative research. The four characteristics potrayed are: order, control, empirical evidence and generalization of scientific method are portrayed. There are limitations in tradition positivistic paradigm, so post-positivistic and naturalistic paradigms emerged.

Chapter 4- "Naturalistic Paradigm" is a conceptual framework to govern the implementation of qualitative research which believes in the complexity of humans. This chapter is a review of the naturalistic paradigm, from historical review to nursing research. Applying "Naturalistic Paradigm" in nursing research, the researcher acts as an instrument, to get a rich and thick description under a natural setting as possible. It allows the researcher to understand the attached meaning of phenomenon and explore more possible associations of it, in instead of verifying a particular hypothesis. As it strongly emphasizes the presence of change, new knowledge and explanation can be generated, and considered useful to improve patient care. In this chapter, the historical review of paradigm shift and characteristics of naturalistic paradigm will be identified first identified. Then, the brief comparison of positivistic and naturalistic paradigm will be discussed. Lastly, the application of naturalistic paradigm in nursing research and its strengths and limitations will be considered.

Chapter 5- This essay is an overview of naturalistic paradigm. The aim of this essay is to obtain an understanding of naturalistic paradigm, from philosophical aspects to its application on research studies. Paradigm is a set of philosophical beliefs on ontology, epistemology and methodology aspects. For naturalistic paradigm, on the ontological aspect, it believes that reality is multiple and subjectively constructed. On the epistemological aspect, it believes that knowledge is created and obtained from an interactive process. On the methodology aspect, it usually associates with qualitative method which emphasizes on collecting narrative information. Naturalistic paradigm emerged from critique toward the traditional research paradigm, positivist paradigm. Therefore, it is a contradicting paradigm towards positivism. Naturalistic and positivist paradigm are two major research paradigms which are often associated with qualitative and quantitative studies, respectively. By contrasting, these two paradigms, it identifies the strength of naturalistic paradigm on addressing research which is sensitive to humanness, such as anthropological and sociological studies. Naturalistic paradigm can be applied y on research studies, from formulating queries y to reporting research findings. Therefore, it is important to understand research paradigm before conducting research.

Chapter 6- Research design is the guide map for the researcher to find out the answer to the research question and it is the most important planning stage in the research process. This article focuses on the selection of the research design with examples of clinical research. Before studying various research designs, criteria of good research designs are discussed to let the novice researcher understand the elements and considerations in order to answer the research question in-depth, effectively and efficiently. Two main research design approaches, quantitative and qualitative research studies y are discussed with their strengths and limitations and implications in nursing and healthcare research.

Chapter 7- Quantitative research is a numerical form of objective presentation. This paper focuses on the different types of research designs in which a nursing researcher would manipulate the entire picture into the quantitative research study. Each research designs has ve its own characteristics as well as pros and cons. It depends on how the research is structured and organized in a systematic ways for setting, sample or other variables that involved in the study.

Chapter 8- There are many types of data collection methods in quantitative research. Data collection is of utmost important in the research process since it can cause a chain of problems if a wrong data collection method is used. Inappropriate sampling and irrelevant data and information will be collected if a wrong data collection method is employed. Therefore, this paper aims to introduce you to the importance of data collection in the research process. After knowing the importance of data collection, this paper will further discuss a type of data collection method – survey – used in quantitative research method. The second part of this paper will introduce you to some optimal questions needed to know before using a survey, and the different variables used in a survey and different types of surveys. Advantages and disadvantages of each type of survey are also discussed in this paper. Finally, Tthe paper finally will briefly explain the recent trend of using Internet survey as a powerful data collection tool.

Chapter 9- Sampling is the process of selecting individuals that represent the population, so that the result obtained from a study can be generalized to that population. This paper focuses on and compares the probability and non-probability sampling strategies used in the quantitative research. Although simple random sampling is said to be the gold standard for quantitative studies, it is rarely adopted due to its cost and complexity. Other modified forms such as stratified sampling, cluster sampling, and systemic sampling are used instead. Though quantitative studies focus on the generalizability of the findings, which the probability sampling can fulfill, non-probability sampling is common in nursing researches. Therefore, it is very important to understand the rationales behind both probability and non-probability samplings in order to decide whether the findings of a study can be applied to a specific group of people. In addition to the kinds of sampling techniques, sample size, sampling error and sampling bias will be briefly discussed as well. This aims to provide a detailed picture of the sampling procedure in the quantitative research.

Chapter 10- Research is a way to generate knowledge, theories and validate the existing knowledge and theories to meet need the current needs of heath system (Panacek and Thompson, 2007). A precise and systematic design of sampling is of paramount importance t to ensure the generalizability and representativeness of the population being studied. There are two main types of sampling: probability sampling which includes simple random sampling, systematic sampling, stratified sampling and cluster sampling; and non-probability sampling which includes convenience sampling, snowball sampling, quota sampling and purposing sampling. In this paper, the application, advantages and disadvantages of each type of sampling will be discussed. The importance of selecting sampling strategies, its utilization, effects on the generalizability and representativeness of the studied population are also discussed.

Chapter 11- This essay notifies the significance of the stage of data collection within the research process. It collects the former theory and the latter practice. The data collected can be classified into two types: quantitative and qualitative. Quantitative data collection is believed to be easier for a fresh researcher. Various quantitative data collection methods are introduced and they are either standardized or non-standardized. The standardized collection methods are well-structured with a high guarantee of reliability. While the non-standardized one, including surveys and questionnaires, measurement scales and biophysiologic measures in nursing research, is more flexible to be adapted to the research approach,. Ttheir strengths are summarized. At last, three important ethical issues should be considered during the collection process.

Chapter 12- Hypothesis testing is the root of scientific research. In quantitative research, statistics are used to accept or reject the null hypothesis in order to answer research questions. In nursing research, statistical tests are often used to analyze the data. There are two main types of statistical tests: parametric and non-parametric tests. The uses and evaluation of these statistical tools are controversial yet necessary. In this paper, differences among parametric and non-parametric tests are depicted, examples and applications in nursing research are illustrated and the evaluation of statistical testing and its interpretation are discussed.

Chapter 13- This essay is a review of the different approaches to quantitative analysis. The aim of this essay is to explain the ideas behind different quantitative analysis methods used in research and through this, explore the differences in the three different approaches, namely, univariate analysis, bivariate analysis and multivariate analysis. With an understanding of these three approaches, a researcher would be able to grasp the distinctiveness of these analyses, the purpose of these analyses and the attainment that these analyses can bring about. Only with a thorough appreciation of these analyses would a researcher be able to plan for the type of methods to use and utilize the quantitative analysis tools well to produce meaningful results. This essay would also include the application of these approaches, in particular the increasingly popular combination of the univariate analysis and multivariate analysis to attempt to explore what these approaches can bring about to the researcher.

Chapter 14- Validity is important in nursing research since it can be used to determine whether the findings of the research are valid or not. The valid findings are valuable in further research studiesy and nursing development. This paper provides some basic information about validity in quantitative research studiesy including some common types of validity and the threats to external and internal validity. In addition, several methods that are used to establish validity are discussed and the criteria in critiquing validity are also mentioned in this paper.

Chapter 15- Quantitative research is a numerical data collection method aimeds at establishing or proving empirical causality between variables. It helps to provide scientific findings for application to the existing clinical problems and for nursing practice improvement. Validity plays an essential role in quantitative research because it ensures the ability of measuring instrument ins reflecting the variables and measuring the concepts of interest accurately. In simple words, validity means the relevance and accuracy of the research. This essay highlights the importance of validity in quantitative nursing research by examining each type of validity, evaluating their purposes and identifying ways to establish them. Choice of validity selection is also discussed, which is made by the researcher basing on the characteristics of target population and measuring instrument, and the availability of a judgmental panel and other comparable validated tools. It is concluded that validity is of high importance in quantitative nursing research. Without establishing validity, the research results generated would possibly be prone to be criticismzed and therefore, spoiling the researcher's effort in conducting it.

Chapter 16- In clinical settings, it is commonly using quantitative approach in conducting nursing research is commonly used. Ssince it is a simpler, faster, more feasible, objective and systematic way to generate data with a goal to obtain findings that help to evaluate the current nursing interventions and enhances better nursing care in the clinical system. Different data collection instruments are used in this type of research. The degree of reliability and validity of the instruments are the two essential issues in ensuring the degree of accuracy of the outcome. This paper will mainly focus on one of the issues – "Reliability". An overview of the quantitative nursing research is first provided, and "Reliability" is defined. Then, a discussion in related to the importance of testing reliability is given. Finally, two commonly used examples of reliability tests: test– retest reliability and interrater reliability are provided.

Chapter 17- Various research literature authors mention many reliability tests to be done before using an instrument in a research. However, most of them do not explain the situations and limitations in using them so that many new researchers are confused when trying to estimate the reliability of the instrument. In this article, a comprehensive review on literature about reliability of nursing research is done to explain the principles of using different reliability tests and the limitations of using these tests. Using a suitable reliability test for the instrument of a research can increase the efficiency to start carrying out a research.

Chapter 18- Qualitative research allows finding out the detailed information from the human society. It includes various approaches such as phenomenology, ethnography, case study and grounded theory. Each of them has their own characteristics to contribute to different research problems and objectives. Familiarizing with different types of research and choosing the most appropriate one for the research is important. This essay introduces the qualitative research and phenomenology, ethnography, case study and grounded theory based on the literature review. In addition, the authors will also express their preference of one research method - ethnography. This essay aims at providing a brief introduction about the qualitative research for who may be the first time to encountering qualitative research for the first time. The authors hope qualitative research will become your friend and you would like to know it more.

Chapter 19- Qualitative interviewing is a way of finding out what others feel and think about their worlds. The authors need to get in- depth information from the interviewees for analysis in qualitative research. A improper informant would speaks superficially or exaggerates the real experience for the sake of holding the researcher's attention and they may be unwilling to trust the interviewer and reveal his or her true feelings. Therefore, it is important to know how to choose the right people to interview who can provide credible information. Clear principles are important to guide the authors to choose proper informants. Purposive sampling and Ttheoretical sampling are often used in qualitative research. They have different criteria. Purposive sampling generally selects informants within extreme situations as for certain characteristics or informants with a wide range of situations in order to maximize variation (Gobo, 2004), while theoretical sampling selects groups or categories to study on the basis of their relevance to research questions and theoretical position, and most importantly, the explanation or account which the authors are developing (Mason, 1996). Regardless of the type of sample employed, informants must be selected or carefully chosen according to specific qualities (Agar, 1980; Hammersley & Atkinson, 1983; Morse, 1991)

Chapter 20- Qualitative research is an objective and systematic approach to explore attitudes, behaviors and experiences via personal interviews or focus groups. These methods only consist of a small sample size. Qualitative research is commonly used in nursing to understand patients care. This paper focuses on whether qualitative research can generalize. Generalizability refers to applying a result from one sample to another sample. Philosophies of both quantitative and qualitative research arend discussed because the issue of generalizability should be traced back to the fundamental issues. Under the scope of the qualitative research, generalizing from a sample to a population is not the first priority. Instead it provides ways to understand human beings and social phenomenon. Since generalizability is rooted from the quantitative research, naturalists argue that it is inappropriate to evaluate the qualitative findings by generalizability. Other naturalists suggest that using transferability to evaluate whether one finding can be used in another population. Transferability is similar to generalizability but requires thick descriptions of the qualitative research. Thick descriptions include clear details of research design, site, sampling, data collection and data analysis method. A paper is evaluated in terms of the transferability, which demonstrates the generalizing power of a qualitative research.

Chapter 21- Qualitative research is a method of inquiry to gather an in-depth understanding of human behavior and reasons governed by the researcher's interpretation. It is traditionally used in social science, and is increasingly recognized and valued in its unique place in nursing disciplines as highlighted by many. With the continuous raising of the problems of objectivity and the validity of qualitative research, this paper aims to focus on technical rigour: the researcher's role in maintaining credibility in trustworthiness. The role of the researcher influences on the internal validity (credibility) in qualitative research in several areas. Both diverse philosophical belief values of qualitative einquiry, as well as different roles of researchers during the research process will be discussed in detail. Finally, recommendations for researchers are suggested in order to provide a guide for them to conduct trustworthiness research papers in the future.

Chapter 22- The significance of a correct research design and the elements of research design for a new researcher to consider when deciding the research approach for a specific study will be discussed in this paper. It is crucial for new researchers to have the above knowledge to maximize the validity of the study. The objective of the paper is to discuss and compare two research designs: descriptive correlational design and mixed method design. Research studies that are conducted using one of these research designs will be chosen as an example to demonstrate the purpose of choosing that particular design with the associated topic. Moreover, the advantages and disadvantages of the research design will be discussed.

Chapter 23- Ethical issues are increasingly reviewed by different institutions across the world, with greater engagement with these processes occurring now (Council for International Organizations of Medical Sciences & World Health Organization, 2002; UNAIDS, 2007; World Medical Association, 2000). Conflicts between the goal of science and the need to protect rights and welfare of human research participants result in the center of ethical tension in clinical research (Derenzo & Moss, 2006); however, some other ethical issues addressing the integrity of clinical research should not be ignored. When even one part of a research project is questionable or conducted unethically, the integrity of the entire project is called into question (Derenzo & Moss, 2006). Thus, it is important for the authors to understand the rationale behind ethical principles in doing research. Based on the evidence of unethical research conducted in the past, this paper would outline different codes issued. Then some ethical principles required for clinical research would be discussed and would be followed by illustrations on the importance of addressing ethical issues properly and sincerely in clinical research. Although the paper would not cover all ethical issues or protocol sections, it aims to assist researchers doing clinical research to be more familiar with ethical considerations.

In: Nursing Research: A Chinese Perspective
Editor: Zenobia C. Y. Chan

ISBN: 978-1-61209-833-3
©2011 Nova Science Publishers, Inc.

Chapter I

Historical Development to Nursing Research

Y. K. Chan and Zenobia C. Y. Chan
The Hong Kong Polytechnic University, China

Summary

There is no doubt that nursing research plays an important role on the development of nursing care. Nursing care have been developed into evidence-based practice and research studies is therefore a must, which will provide more evidence in nursing practice and thus can evaluate the effectiveness of nursing care provided. Understanding the history of the nursing research could help us to realize the development of the nursing research and its relationship with other aspects of nursing such as the development of nursing education and change in nursing role. Research will help to build up a scientific knowledge-base for nursing practice which includes health promotion, protection and prevention from illness, optimization of health condition for not only the people who are critically ill, but also for those who are healthy thus, providing holistic care to everyone. Through research, a cost-effective health care system can be developed and also provide an ensuring standard of nursing care.

Introduction

Nursing care is holistic, concerning the environmental impact to individuals, psychological status of individuals, nutritional status of individuals, social status of individuals and physiological well-being. By conducting research, nursing interventions can be improved and thus can help individuals to achieve their optimal functioning and self-care. Hence, Nursing Research is one of the key elements for nursing development.

Burns and Grove (2001) has defined that nursing research is "a scientific process that validates and refines existing knowledge and generates new knowledge that directly and indirectly influences nursing practice" (p. 4). Nursing research is a method of obtaining knowledge to strengthen new ideas in clinical nursing practice, enhance nursing education and nursing administration by describing the relationship between phenomena. Nursing research can be conducted in a systematic and objective manner through repeated trial and error in experiments, personal nursing experiences and literature reviews. The development of nursing research is directly influenced by nursing models, nurse role and nursing education and vice versa. The relationship of nursing research, nursing models, nursing role and education are studied as follow.

Nursing Models and Nursing Research

An Environmental Adaptation theory by Florence Nightingale mentions that nurses should make observations for patients and make documentation in a systematic way and use statistical data to illustrate the findings. Her advice is followed by nurses until now. Nurses are recommended to explore new knowledge and validate the trustfulness of nursing theory and practice during the process of data collection and analysis of data. This helps nursing practice to grow into a standardized and evidence-based practice. In this way, nurses can review patient's records, make accurate clinical judgment and hence, have a close monitor of the patient's health status (Laing, 2002). Evidence-based practice also facilitates the process of nursing research by the use of scientific information from randomized clinical trials (Long & Harrison, 1996; Mion, 1998; Rochon, Dikinson & Gordon, 1997). The topic of research now is also influenced by the theory, which one of the focuses is to find out the change in the environmental setting that can improve the health of the public and prevent communicable disease (Andrist, Nicholas & Wolf, 2006). Her theories also contribute a lot to the research topic, her theory offers a guideline for research and a framework for generating knowledge and new ideas (McEwen & Wills, 2002).

The adaption's model by Callista Roy that mainly focuses on the outcome. There are four adaptive modes; physiological mode, self-concept mode, role function mode and interdependence mode (McQuiston & Webb, 1995). Physiological mode is the assessment of a person in adapting to physiological needs. Self-concept mode is the ability to recognize self and it is a sense of unity. Role function mode is the assessment of how a person behaves in different roles which means to determine the social life of a person. Interdependence mode is the assessment that is used to determine whether a person has the sense of security within a relationship. One example of research that uses the framework of Roy's Adaption's model is *Changes in functional status after childbirth* (Tulman, Fawcett, Groblewski & Silverman, 1990).The researcher used the model as a framework to raise research question, it also provides a gateway for a clear explanation of the interrelationship between modes.

The Neuman Systems model by Betty Neuman that mainly focuses on the reaction of clients when facing stressors in the environment and the related nursing intervention. In the theory, she mentions that a client may be defined as an individual, family, a group or community. The client is treated as any system that contains the energy to interact with stressors in environment. Her model is used in wide variety of clinical settings, for example, used as a guide for setting up interviews that assess stressors of the client in a research study (McQuiston & Webb, 1995). Five variables are identified in the theory. They included physiological, psychological, developmental, sociocultural and spiritual variables. Her theory can also be a guide to set up a hypothesis that is to set up the assumption to find out the relationship between client and stressors. One example of the research that is done using the Neuman's System Model namely, *"Neuman's System model for Nursing Practice as a Conceptual Framework for a Family Assessment"* (Herrick & Goddykoontz, 1989). In this research, the researcher conducts interviews with all of the family members to assess the types and sources of stressors on the family system.

Hildegard E. Peplau mentions that nurses should prepare themselves to have multiple roles, as caregiver, researcher and expert. The Nature of Nursing by Virginia Henderson also mentions a qualified nurse should be responsibility for validating and improving the effectiveness of the nursing procedure. By conducting research, nurses are able to show their value in the medical field and are able to enrich their knowledge base. The graduate programs are established in the twentieth century due to the increasing demand of more advanced education and more specific clinical practice by nurses. There is a remarkable change in the education level of nursing from only a diploma certificate to a graduate or master certificate holder. Due to the change in the nurse role, more nurses have changed their role from caregiver in the front line into researcher, teacher and even counselor. At the same time, nurses are well-equipped with knowledge on theory and from other disciplines such as psychological and pharmacology, their ability to conduct research studies become higher. The perception of people in women's roles and culture difference also influences the development of the nurse role. In the past, it is mainly a male- dominant society that women should not play an important role in society and women should be less educated than men. Nowadays, many people suggest that there should be equality between men and women, hence, women have a chance to chase for knowledge.

Nurse Role and Nursing Research

Nurse role plays two important parts for the nursing research. Externally, the recognition of the nursing research is dependent on the nurse role in the society. Internally, the role of nurse should be more than a caregiver. Nurses should treat research as part of her job duty and responsibility. The contribution extent of the nurse has a direct impact on nursing research development.

Regarding the nurse role in society, its status was highly increased by Virginia Henderson during the Victorian era. She mentions that nurses should have a unique function. In the past, women are stereotyped as fragile, weak and they have a traditional submissive role. Women should maintain the harmony of the family and their works are restricted while men should go out and gain money for the family. During the period of the Victorian era, nurses are women and this stereotype of women should not be present, thus there is a need to reform the image of women. By playing an important role in treating illness, the society begins to recognize that nurses should have a unique role and in this way, the image of women has been changed. In the Crimean War, the mortality rate of British soldiers drops under the care of Florence Nightingale (McQuiston & Webb, 1995; Zerwekh & Claborn,

2009). Her great success has brought nurses into a unique function which makes nursing research more well-recognized and respected.

Other than raising the status of a nurse in society, nurses should also recognize their roles on the development nursing research. They should understand and identify the essence and benefits of performing the nursing research. In the past, many of the nurses were educated in the hospital-based nursing school, their study and learning is mainly focus on the practical parts. However, the situation has been changed because of the rapid development of medical technology and knowledge. The education model of nurses has been switched to evidence-based practice. Moreover, nursing research is also put as part of the standard nursing curriculum in order to facilitate the professional development of the role and facilitate the nurse to manage and handle their daily works.

Many nursing specialties have been developed such as pediatric, mental health and gerontological nursing due to the need for a higher quality of care. Thus, nurses need a more advanced education and training. Nurses can also absorb knowledge by a self-searching information technique and trial-and–error method. Self- searching technique is to search information related to diagnosis, intervention and come through theory review. Trial-and-error method is the repeated testing on the effectiveness of intervention on a specific diagnosis. These are two techniques commonly used in research. Research will enable the provision of more advanced care, higher quality and more cost-effective nursing care.

Nursing Education and Nursing Research

The successes of Florence Nightingale in infection control and statistical research have been highlighted even until now. She was the first to identify nurses needs to be well-educated with theory and their need to skillful with practice In 1860, Florence Nightingale established the School of Nursing in St. Thomas's Hospital in London, and it was the first secular nursing school in the world (McEwen & Wills, 2002). She aimed at providing education to hospital nurses so that those nurses can be the educator for other nurses. Nurses were educated and trained under her theory. (Zerwekh & Claborn, 2009). Many nursing schools were then established based on her concepts of education. Most of the nursing schools were hospital-based and provided training in the clinical skills (Tomey & Alligood, 2006). This hospital-based education is contrasted with todays university-based education and hospital-based education is more focused on clinical skill training where university-based education is more focused on academic achievement (Barr & Sines, 2009).

Since the Second World War, medical, surgery and clinical knowledge have developed rapidly. However, a knowledge gap was developed between the health care parties – doctors and nurses is one of the typical cases. To overcome this gap, nurses are required to conduct research and study to strengthen their nursing knowledge so as to facilitate their daily works which lead sto an increase in the demand of high level education nurse. Since the 1950s, the US has started to establish the doctoral program for nursing and the development was sped up. From the 1950s to 1980s, the numbers of doctoral programs were increased from 2 to 29 with more than a 1400% increase with nearly one new program increase each year on average (Freshwater & Bishop, 2004).

Nevertheless, the education system is still not capable to support the development of nursing. In the 1980s, only about 2,400 nurses had studied at the doctoral level, which is less than 0.2% of the nurse's population (Anderson, 2000). Therefore, there is a revolution change in nursing education in the United States from the 1980s to 1990s. The number of doctoral programs has been increased from 29 to 70 with a 240% increase within 10 years (Freshwater & Bishop, 2004). On average, 4 new doctoral programs were developed per year. On the other hand, the amount of nursing research was increased significantly from the 1950s to 1990s. The change in educational preparation from diploma degree to masters or even a doctoral degree, will provide a higher quality of research studies because nurses become more knowledgeable and have a more diverse interest in researching in different health aspect. Professionalism of nursing is also enhanced by conducting a research with higher quality.

Until now, nursing education leads to several different degrees and specialties, including post-graduate work, and nursing theory has evolved to meet the challenges of this diversification and increasing professionalization. Therefore, nursing research and nursing education is inter-related and they influence each other. Nursing research would require the support from nursing education – talents and experts. On the other hand, education would also require the support from nursing research –the latest knowledge and skills.

Conclusion

Owing to the above mentioned, research, education, nursing role and theory are interrelated. In order to manage the increasing demand for a high level of education requirement, nurses should also have a role not only as a caregiver but also as a researcher. Nursing is a career that requires one to enrich her knowledge from time to time. Knowledge development is cumulative and nurses should obtain new knowledge through conducting research continuously. When studying for a master and/or doctoral degree, nurses should be well-prepared for research. Research is a part of showing the intelligence, accountability and responsiveness of a nurse. Hence, there is a need to continue research in the future .

Author's Background

Chan Yik Kam, a year two student who is studying Master of Nursing in the Hong Kong Polytechnic University. (Email: niriko_chan@hotmail.com)

References

Anderson, C.A. (2000). Current Strengths and Limitations of Doctoral Education in Nursing; are we prepare for the future. *Journal of Professional Nursing*, 16(4), 191-200.

Andrist, L.C., Nicholas, P.K. & Wolf, K.A. (2006). *A History of Nursing Ideas*. Jones and Bartlett Publishers Canada.

Barr, O. & Sines, D. (2009). The development of the generalist nurse within pre-registration nurse education in the UK: some points for consideration. *Nurse Education Today.* 4, 274–277.

Burns, N. & Grove, S. K. (2001). *The practice of nursing research: Conduct, critique and utilization (4th Ed.).* Philadelphia: Saunders.

Chaska, N.L. (2001). *The Nursing Profession: Tomorrow and beyond.* California: Sage.

Forchuk, C. (1990). Peplau's Inter-personal theory. In A. Baumann,N. Johnson & D. Atai-Otaong, *Decision-making in psychiatric and psychosocial nursing* (p.22-23). Toronto B. C. Decker.

Freshwater, D. & Bishop, V. (2004). *Nursing Research in Context: Appreciation, Application & Professional Development.* Palgrave Macmillan.

Halloran, E.J. (1995). *A Virginia Henderson Reader: Excellence in Nursing.* Springer Publishing Company

Herrick, C.A. & Goddykoontz, L. (1989). Neuman's System model for Nursing Practice as a Conceptual Framework for a Family Assessment. *Journal of Child Adolescent Psychiatric Mental Health Nursing,* 2(2), 61-67.

Joel, L.A. (2003). *Kelly's Dimensions of Professional Nursing* (9th Ed.) USA:McGraw-hill.

Laing, K. (2002). The benefits and challenges of the computerized electronic medical record. *Gastroenterol Nursing.*25(2)41-45.

Long, A. & Harrison,S. (1996). Evidence-based decision making. *Health Service Journal,* 106(5486 Health Manage Guide), 1-12.

McEwen, M. & Wills, E.M. (2007). *Theoretical basis for Nursing(2nd Ed.).* Philadelphia PA: Lippincott Williams & Wikins.

McQuiston, C.M. & Webb, A.A. (1995). *Foundations of Nursing Theory: Contributions of 12 Key Theorists.* California: Sage.

Mertens, E. I., Halfens, R. J. G., Dietz, E., Scheufele, R. & Dassen, T. (2008). Pressure ulcer risk screening in hospitals and nursing homes with a general nursing assessment tool: evaluation of the care dependency scale. *Journal of Evaluation in Clinical Practice,* 14(6), 1018-1025.

Mion, L.C. (1998). Evidence-based health care practice. *Journal of Gerontological Nursing,* 24(12), 5-6.

Neuman, B.M. (2011). *The Neuman Systems model (5th ed.).* Boston: Pearson.

Nieswiadomy, R.M. (2008). *Foundations of Nursing Research.* (5th Ed.) USA: Prentice Hall.

Peplau, H.E. (1952). *Inter-personal relations in nursing.* New York:G.P.Putnam.

Peplau, H.E. (1962). Inter-personal techniques: The crux of psychiatric nursing. *American Journal of Nursing,* 62, 50-54.

Rochon, P.A., Dikinson, E. & Gordon, M. (1997). The Cochrane field in health care of older people: Geriatric medicine's role in collaboration. *Journal of the American Geriatrics Society,* 45(2), 241-243.

Tomey, A. M. & Alligood, M. R. (2006). *Nursing Theorists and their Work (6th ed.).* Mosby: St. Louis.

Tulman, L., Fawcett, J., Groblewski, L. & Silverman, L. (1990). Changes in functional status after childbirth. *Nursing Research.* 39,70-75

Zerwekh, J. & Claborn, J.C. (2009). *Nursing Today:transition and trends(6th ed.).*Canada: Saunders   Elsevier.

In: Nursing Research: A Chinese Perspective
Editor: Zenobia C. Y. Chan

ISBN: 978-1-61209-833-3
©2011 Nova Science Publishers, Inc.

Chapter II

Overview on Positivist Paradigm and its Application in Nursing Research

P. S. Wong and Zenobia C. Y. Chan
The Hong Kong Polytechnic University, China

Summary

This essay provides a brief review of positivist paradigm. The aim of this paper gives a basic understanding of positivist paradigm, the characteristics and its influences to nursing research. Positivist paradigm is commonly used in research that acquires knowledge from observing the fact in the natural world objectively with scientific measurement. And iIt is dominant and has great influences to nursing research development. In this essay, the historical and philosophical aspects will be first overviewed first. Next, the ontology, epistemology and methodology in philosophical aspects will be described briefly, and the characteristics of the paradigm are followed. Finally, the relationship between positivist paradigm and nursing research development will be discussed as the conclusion.

Introduction

Nursing development has been influenced by many factors like the challenge of profession by traditional professional disciplines like medicine. In an attempt to develop a knowledge base as a profession, the importance of nursing research development has awoken awaked and the quality of nursing practice is kept enhancing for many years. Back to the history of nursing research development, positivist paradigm had become a dominant approach throughout the process. Even up to now, nursing researches cannot be replaced by other corresponding, newly- developed beliefs like naturalistic paradigm. Although there is an conflict that many researchers argued that the development of the research has a got great impact by positivistic paradigm, which just focuses on using scientific methods to separate nurses from the 'real world', it and contradicts to the humanistic approach of nursing. This controversial issue is still carrying on and no definite conclusion is found. It shows that positivist paradigm has somewhere to "live". The development of nursing research causes a great impact in nursing discipline and nursing practice as it helps the establishment of specific knowledge, reinforcement of the position in the profession and evaluation of nursing practice in care.

Therefore, in this essay, the development of the positivism starting from its history, is briefly described. The definitions and concepts of each term including positivism, paradigm, positivist paradigm and quantitative research follow to be shown in order to establish the basic idea for research design before implementation. Next, the relationship of positivist paradigm and nursing discipline and nursing development respectively, are also discussed. Eventually, the benefit by using the paradigm in the nursing area and its limitations are described as well in the essay.

Historical Development of Positivism

Positivism was developed more than a hundred years ago in western countries. The history of positivism might be extended from ancient times to the present. Before the 19th century, empiricists and sensationalists commonly believed that all knowledge comes from experiences and started to use introspection to explain natural events in the social world, but it was examined by their private experiences only (Hesse & Leavy, 2011). In the natural world, physical phenomena are governed by scientific laws and result in a pattern that such patterned social reality can then be predicted, and potentially controlled, from the view of positivists (Hesse & Leavy, 2011). Therefore, in the social science, positivism, which was first promoted by a French philosophist called Auguste Comte (1798-1857), started to be used to equating knowledge with empirical and public observations in order to increase the rigor and truthfulness in social science (Hergenhahn, 2005). As a result, the rationale of positivism was developed which caused profound influence as a very idea to subsequent research development in all kinds of disciplines. And it became omes dominated and applied through the method of quantitative research in sociology, psychology, education as well as in nursing discipline. Therefore, in the following section, the introduction of positivism is going to be described, paradigm is followed, and the integration of the above two terms and the quantitative research are also introduced. The characteristics in each of them are briefly shown in Table 1 as below.

Table 1. The characteristics of each term

Terms	Characteristics
Positivism	A belief to present the natural fact into knowledge through scientific measurement
Paradigm	A framework to gather and show all relevant concepts
Positivist paradigm	The integration of positivism and paradigm to review the world objectively
Quantitative research	A method to test or examine the hypothesis under positivist paradigm.

Overview of Positivism, Positivistic Paradigm and Quantitative Research

According to Comte, he stated that Ppositivism proposed that e reality and truth in the natural world can be determined through empirical observations (Hergenhahn, 2005). It also refers to a belief that the researchers try to find out things or discover empirical facts through scientific ways with careful measurement (Edwards, 1998). Besides, positivism is also the framework of the natural sciences, like biology and chemistry, that are presented in the form of scientific laws and characterized via laboratory or experimental research (Norwood, 2010). Therefore, positivism is a belief that tries to show the knowledge or fact in the natural world to become presentable through experiments and numbers.

The term paradigm is defined as a pattern or example that provides an abstract view of different concepts, perspective of a discipline, or a set of beliefs to explain a complex process, idea or set of data effectively which is accepted by most scientists, and is also described as "general scientific perspectives and traditions", as the development of nursing science is based on various research traditions and different perspectives used to solve problems in nursing disciplines (Monti & Tingen, 1999). In research, paradigm plays a very important role in the science community as it gives a general orientation directing scientists to do research (Monti & Tingen, 1999). Thus, it would acts as a framework to guide scientists on how to resolves the problem and conduct in the correct direction, so that scientists can follow the same rule and have unified standards for scientific practices if they share the same paradigm based on the ontological and epistemological assumptions. As a result, many nursing scientists use the paradigm as a guideline throughout their research processes like research design, problem investigations, as well as methodology.

Therefore, positivist paradigm used in quantitative research refers to the objective view of the reality or truth by using traditional scientific methods under the assumption that the process is never affected by historical, social or cultural context (Bonell, 1999). This perspective forms the basis to direct the researchers to investigate, study and find out the meanings of the knowledgeable reality and the development of the universal principles, laws and outcomes through scientific ways, like experiments and surveys without personal bias. Therefore, it is known as the positivist-empiricist paradigm (Doordan, 1998).

While qQuantitative research is a kind s of research studying different variables, which are pre-selected and defined by researchers, and emphasizes to gather all empirical evidences from the root of the objective reality directly or indirectly through senses (Norwood, 2010). The cause-to-effect relationships can be established after the ordered process in the ways of data collection with statistical analysis. As the research is scientific- and mathematical- based, the rigor of the research is strongly reflected.

Referring to the Table 1 with the introduction of the above terms, the following question that comes to the mind would then be the relationship about them with the research establishment and the application in the research aspect. Hence, infiltrating into the philosophy of paradigm may offer you the answer shown in the following section.

Philosophy of Paradigm (Ontology, Epistemology and Methodology)

Philosophy of paradigm is constituted of ontology, epistemology and methodology which are the inquiries into the conditions of knowledge (Wainwright, 1996). Ontology is defined as what exists, epistemology refers to how we can get to know the knowledge related to those being researched, and methodology means the method we used to acquire this knowledge (Wainwright, 1996, Polit & Beck, 2004). Such concepts can be presented in a more clear way by showing them in to questions. "What kinds of things exist in the world?" refers to ontology; "How do we gain the knowledge of the world?" refers to epistemology (Hughes & Sharrock, 1997). It makes the experience as the foundation of all kinds of knowledge and acts as a complementary of ontology to provide a vision of the knowledge that is accessible through observation (Bryant, 1985).

When the philosophy is applied on the research aspect, it would be linked up with phenomena, positivist paradigm and quantitative research, respectively. For ontology, it would be referred to as the phenomena we experienced or observed , which is pre-exists ed, we experienced or observed in the natural world and pre-selected by the researchers; while epistemology refers to the positivist paradigm which is usually in contrast to a positivist-deductive approach with experimental design, quantitative data and traditional statistical methods (Glinder & Morgan, 2000). And the methodology is the deductive process that emphasizes on discrete but specific concepts or measured with quantitative data information through statistical analysis (Polit & Beck, 2004). Therefore, before getting started with to any research, there are several aspects required to be considered including the existence of the thing decided to be studied and the means on getting to know about it. And then, the method to get the required data or information is followsed. And thus, it revealed that it is a structure and sequence for research design when a research is going to be established. Hence, after such consideration, if positivist paradigm is chosen from the amount of paradigms and as the basis of a research, experimental design involving testing a single, pre-selected hypothesis through a statistical method is used that was labeled as a method of quantitative research.

Characteristics of Positivist Paradigm in Quantitative Research

According to Norwood in 2010, he stated that research involves data collection, data analysis and result interpretation in order to describe, explain, predict and control phenomena depending on the purpose of the researchers, by like either refining or examining the prior knowledge or generating new knowledge. Additionally, he also listed out the several features of research and gave brief explanations to each of them shown namely rigor, reliability and validity, empirical and control. Rigor in the research refers to the manifestation of excellence and accuracy through systematic striving during research study. Reliability and validity are defined as trustworthiness and accuracy shown by the measurement of the research. And empirical refer to things that can be observed or verified through observation from the reality by human senses. The empirical data is collected in an objective ways which absolutely gets rid of any subjective belief or personal biases. Last but not least ss, control is stated as the ability to control the phenomena by the desired outcome. Those features are different among different kinds of researches.

While for the characteristics of positivist paradigm, in the accordance of the explanation from Monti & Tingen in 1999, positivist paradigm aims to share values, assumptions or knowledge pre-existing ed in the natural world or reality and being observed in an the objective point of view and described via a statistical method with numbers. During the research process, those things being studied would not be interfere ed with the phenomena and would be presented in mathematical ways. The paradigm adheres closely with the philosophy of the method and easily identified the values and beliefs behind the study.

Hence, when positivist paradigm is chosen and applied in the research, this method is then highly rigorous as it integrates d both characteristics described in the previous two paragraphs. And it is also empirical enough to equally ized utilized the knowledge without involving any subjective bias from its past experiences or pre-supposed values. Besides, the as cause-to-effect relationship is mostly investigated, examined or verified for finding out the solutions of the problem or factors triggering the phenomena as the final outcome of the research. The control in this kind of research is correspondingly higher than the others, which means that the phenomena can then be predicted through the outcomes of the research. However, for reliability and validity, it is difficult to show how much it is at the beginning stage of constructing the research, but it is relatively better than the research involving the hermeneutic method such as behavior research.

Therefore, based on such significant and unique characteristics, the following section is going to discuss the impact of positivist paradigm brought to the nursing research development. In the first place, some background is given which briefly describes the historical development of nursing research followed by and the influence of it would then follow.

Paradigm Influences to the Evolution of Nursing Research Development

Since the time of Nightingale, being 150 years before, nursing had been aware of developing its own theoretical knowledge with applying it to nursing practice (Kirkevold, 1997). However, there was no idea on how to make it at the beginning. In the early stage of theoretical ideas, they were derived from personal knowledge, clinical observation and philosophical thinking (Kirkevold, 1997) and thus, the research used at that moment was mainly focused on nursing practice but less useful for guiding nursing research (Hinshaw, 1999). which That leaded to traditional nursing interventions that relied on tradition as a source of knowledge for safe security and saving time-saving (Norwood, 2010).

Meanwhile, nursing was facing challenges from other prior professional disciplines like medicine which is a that profession of discipline was justified by the credibility of its research. Hence, nursing was required to establish its own scientific research and specialized knowledge base for professional seeking simultaneously (Wuest, 1994 & Weaver & Olson, 2005). Since the increase of emphasis and urgency on building its own body of knowledge in nursing, the application of positivistic paradigm in nursing research can help it become more of a professional approach (Playle, 1995). Thus, nursing borrowed theories from other disciplines like sociology, whose that their scientific-empirical system had been already developed to meet its practical needs (Meleis, 2007). As a result, the development of nursing research is influenced deeply by that of sociological research that positivist paradigm become dominant throughout the development and reinforced its professional position at the same time.

In nursing science, it is characterized by two predominant paradigms, namely the empiricist and the interpretative, respectively. Here, the former one would be mainly discussed in this paper. As described in the above section, the empiricism focus on verifying the assumption through the senses and the ontological assumption of it would then be the reality found based on it. In tTraditionally, nursing research focused on the context of justification (Monti & Tingen, 1999). Positivism, with using an antiquated view of the universe, believed that the world ran as a machine under the laws of science, and these laws can be discovered or defined so as to explain or predict events in the natural world (Monti & Tingen, 1999). Thus, theories used to describe, predict and prescribe the science are the outcome of the study while ith separating the whole phenomena into components in order to find all possible factors behind it. In fact, science emphasizes on numbers which is a kind of method that o justifies y the validity of the theories or laws. And the purpose of the scientific investigation in nursing is very important because the generalization is the final goal of the study for nursing so that the theories can then be applied on other similar populations. Therefore, personal biases of the researchers should be prevented throughout the study,. While so the methodology associated with the empiricism would then be the scientific method as quantitative research. It emphasizes on the experiment, control, data collection and analysis and the description of results by statistical means (Monti & Tingen, 1999) so that the hypothesis going to be tested can be shown in numerical values, with using statistical methods.

Therefore, the empiricist (positivist) paradigm is necessary for providing explanatory models and the means to either test or generate nursing theories for improving nursing care and predicting the responses of persons under different health stages by investigating the proper reasons behind. Furthermore, the empirical research helps nursing develop ing its own knowledge by examining different kinds of hypotheseis so that nursing interventions can be compared and then produce generalization. Generalizability is very important in empirical research and acts as the final goal of the research (Burn & Grove, 2003, Monti & Tingen, 1999). It provides great benefits to nursing practices and the patients in need s because it allows the hypothesis, like relationships, to be extrapolated to different situations or larger populations.

Therefore, nursing research with using the paradigm provides a scientific process that modifies, validates or re-examines the existing nursing theories and generates new knowledge in order to improve nursing care provided and health care to people in the community. And it also influences nursing practice directly and indirectly because it acts as a guideline and empirical knowledge- base to guide practice and justify the quality of nursing care. Even though the positivist paradigm provides many much contributions to nursing research development, there is more required tthere is not everything round to cover all needs in the application. There must be some limitation found in each method. The limitation of using positivist paradigm in the research will be shown in the following section.

Limitation of Positivist Paradigm

Positivism- used research focuses on studying the knowledge of interest in the objective way, which is a lack of holistic consideration (Weaver & Olson, 2005). Positivism acquires new knowledge or theories by using scientific measurementss and explains the phenomena or meaning mathematically. However, it is difficult to measure or define subjective feeling or spiritual aspects by using numerical expressions such as like lived experiences of the patient, personal perspectives about an issue, and so on (Edwards, 1998). Besides, there may be other potential factors varying the outcome simultaneously or being hidden behind the fact. However, positivist paradigm research based on pre-observed hypothesis may be too narrow to find out all of the possible factors within a research. Though there are some limitations found in the positivist paradigm, it is still dominant in the application to the most of researches in all disciplines.

Conclusion

In this essay, positivist paradigm is introduced in both historical and philosophical ways. With the understanding of the characteristics of the paradigm, the basic idea of positivist paradigm is established which helps the researchers for designing their research. Apart from these, the review of positivist paradigm used for nursing research has allowed us to identify issues that the paradigm still plays a very significant role in nursing research. The powerful support from the long-termed historical development of the paradigm and scientific-based trustworthiness is provided and enhances the confidence of the researchers on the application of the paradigm in nursing research even though they study under the great influences caused by the conflict against the use of a positivist approach. Furthermore, some benefits brought from the usage of the paradigm with nursing disciplinary development are emphasized in the ways of specific knowledge evaluation, professional position maintenance , and the improvement of nursing practice through the application of the paradigm in nursing research.

Author's Background

Wong Pui Shan, Stella, a year two student who is studying Master of Nursing in the Hong Kong Polytechnic University and the Hong Kong Sanatorium Hospital. (Email: stella_wps@yahoo.com.hk)

References

Bonell, C. (1999). Evidence-based nursing: a stereotyped view of quantitative and experimental research could work against professional autonomy and authority. *Journal Of Advanced Nursing*, 30 (1), pp. 18-23

Burns. N., & Grove. S. K. (2003). *Understanding nursing research* (3rd ed.). Saunders Elsevier Inc

Bryant, C. G. A. (1985). *Positivism in social theory and research.* Macmillan Publishers Ltd: London

Doordan, A. M. (1998). *Lippincott's need-to-know: research survival guide.* Lippincott: Philadelphia

Edwards, S. D. (1998). *Philosophical issues in nursing.* Macmillan press Ltd: London Gliner, J. A., & Morgan, G. A. (2000). *Research methods in applied settings: An integrated approach to designs and analysis.* Lawrence Erlbaum Associates Inc:

Hergenhahn, B. R. (2005). *An introduction to the history of psychology* (5th ed.). Thomson Wadswort: USA

Hess, S. N., & Leavy, B. P. (2011). *The practice of qualitative research* (2nd ed.). SAGE Publication Inc: UK

Hinshaw, A. S. (1999). Evolving nursing research traditions: influencing factors. In *Handbook of Clinical Nursing.* Sage Thousand Oaks: USA

Hughes, J., & Sharrock, W. (1997). *The philosophy of social research* (3rd ed.). Addison Wesley Longman Limited: UK

Kirkevold, M. (1997). Integrative nursing research – an important strategy to further the development of nursing science and nursing practice. *Journal of Advanced Nursing, 25,* 977–984.

Meleis, A. I. (2007). *Theoretical nursing: development and progress* (4th ed.). Lippincott Williams & Wilkins: Philadelphia

Monti, E.J., & Tingen, M. S. (1999). Multiple paradigms in nursing science. *Advances In Nursing Science*, 99(6), 21 (4), pp. 64-80

Norwood, S. L. (2010). *Research essentials foundation for edvidence-based practice.* Pearson Education Inc

Nyatanga, L.(2005). Nursing and philosophy of science, *Nurse Education Today.* 25 (8), pp. 670-4

Playle, J. F. (2005). Humanism and positivism in nursing: Contradictions and conflicts. *Journal Of Advanced Nursing*, 22 (5), pp. 979-84

Polit, D. F., & Beck, C. T. (2004). *Nursing research: principles and methods* (7th ed.). Lippincott Williams & Wilkins: Philadelphia

Wainwright, S. P. (1996). A new paradigm for nursing: the potential of realism. *Journal Of Advanced Nursing*, 26 (6), pp. 1262-71

Weaver, K., & Olson, J. K. (2006). Understand paradigms used for nursing research. *Journal Of Advanced Nursing*, 53 (4), pp. 459-6

Wuest, J. (1994). Professionalism and the evolution of nursing as a discipline: a feminist perspective. *Journal of Professional Nursing,* 10, 357–367.

In: Nursing Research: A Chinese Perspective
Editor: Zenobia C. Y. Chan

ISBN: 978-1-61209-833-3
©2011 Nova Science Publishers, Inc.

Chapter III

Understanding Positivistic Paradigm in Nursing Research

Henry W. S. Tam and Zenobia C. Y. Chan
The Hong Kong Polytechnic University, China

Summary

This article demonstrates the positivistic paradigm in nursing discipline. The importance of positivism and paradigm is briefly described. The philosophical assumptions of positivistic paradigm in ontology, epistemology, axiology, rhetorical structure, and methodology are discussed for having a better understanding. A quantitative research example was used for the illustration of assumptions. The Aapplication on positivistic paradigm in research is quantitative research. The four characteristics potrayed are: order, control, empirical evidence and generalization of scientific method are portrayed. There are limitations in tradition positivistic paradigm, so post-positivistic and naturalistic paradigms emerged.

Introduction

Nursing research has grown over the past 100 years from focusing primarily on nursing education to developing a scientific knowledge base for the practice of nursing, for providing optimal nursing care (Dempsey & Dempsey, 2000). Often, the nursing research is classified into quantitative and qualitative research by a methodological point of view. It is because the methodological structure is important in designing the research study, especially data collection and analysis process. It is closer to research practice than paradigm. On the other hand, before undergoing a quantitative or qualitative research, as a researcher, it is better to understand what the rationales and justifications that are behind supporting their work. Research paradigm contains the philosophical assumptions and foundations that provide the ground for research development. Therefore, researchers, from novice to expert level, should fully understand wholly the philosophy of science parameters undergirding their research worldview and academic work (Ponterotto, 2005).

In nursing discipline, there are two major paradigms; the namely positivistic paradigm and the naturalistic paradigm,. Bboth of which have legitimacy for nursing research. The paradigm that dominated nursing research for many years is known as positivism (Pilot & Beck, 2008). Therefore, it is a good to understand and consolidate the essences of positivism and positivistic paradigm not only for reviewing the literatures and but also for conducting the future research. This paper will provide the reader with a basic foundation on positivistic paradigm. It can be divided into four main parts. It starts with the definition of terms including positivism and paradigm. The characteristics, strength and weakness of the paradigm are discussed afterward to present a clearer picture. The paradigmatic application in research and quantitative research are described to show a concrete demonstration. Finally, the current situation and development of positivistic paradigm in the local setting will be discussed.

Positivism

Positivism is thought to have been rooted in the 19th century, which is guided by philosophers like Comte, Mill, Newton, and Locke (Polit & Beck, 2004, p.13). It is an expression of a broader cultural phenomenon, which is referred to as modernism in the humanities. Reflecting the belief that experience accessed through the senses is the only source of factual knowledge. It emphasizes on a rational and scientific way of thinking. Science was viewed as the only repository of all human knowledge with a role of formulating laws and theories, making prediction and controlling of phenomena based on observation (Powers & Knapp, 2006).

Positivistic Paradigm

A paradigm can be defined as a "set of interrelated assumptions about the social world which provides a philosophical and conceptual framework for the organized study of that world" (Filstead, 1979, p. 34).

In conducting a scientific inquiry, the philosophical assumptions, goals and purposes of a particular mode of inquiry are the guidelines for the researcher in the selection of tools, instruments, participants, and methods used in the study (Denzin & Lincoln, 2000), which is known as a research paradigm. Paradigm is like a model and which is "similar to an action plan that describes work to be done in a discipline and fames an orientation within which the work will be accomplished" (Powers & Knapp, 1995, p.188)

The primary goal of positivistic research is a reasoning deduction that leads to the prediction and control of phenomena.

The Assumption Components of Positivistic Paradigm

The philosophy of science parameters including ontology, epistemology, axiology, rhetorical structure and methodology of positivistic paradigm are discussed in the following paragraphs. Within paradigm, each parameter has gets a concern and which can be clarified by a question. An research paper was used as an example for illustration.

Ontology

Ontology concerns the nature of reality. It can be addressed by the question: What is the nature of reality? The answer from positivists is realism or objectivsm. Positivists contend that there is one true reality, which can be apprehended, identifiable and measurable (Ponterotto, 2005). For example, Smith (2006) conducted a research on the effect of hypnotherapy upon a health-related quality of life (HRQoL) in patients with irritable bowel syndrome (IBS). In the studies, the statuses of the subjects were assessed and measured by the item measurement theory.

Epistemology

Epistemology is concerned with the relationship between the inquirer and those being researched. It can be addressed by: what is the relationship of the researcher to that being researched? It is because objective reality is the belief of positivists. The positivists doing the research would try to avoid their personal beliefs and bias contaminating the phenomena obtained in the studies. They are independent from the subject. It is to prevent any influences that exerted from the investigator in the research. Smith (2006) didn't have interaction with the subjects. He only had the pre-assessment, intervention and post-assessment with the subjects.

Axiology

Axiology concerns the role of researcher values in the scientific process. It can be addressed by the question: what is the role of values in the research?

In positivistic paradigm research, value-free research is conducted when the beliefs of the researcher do not have any effect on the way in which the data is collected or analyzed. The experience and beliefs, such as like religious, of the researcher should be not be imposed when the research is collected. It can be noticed in the Smith (2006) research paper.

Rhetorical Structure

Rhetoric refers to the language used to present the procedures and results of research to one's intended audience. It can be addressed by the question: what is the language and voice to be used in the research? Positivists act as objectivity, with and a detached and emotionally neutral research role, presenting in a precise and scientific manner (Ponterotto, 2005). Smith (2006) uses 'patient' or 'subject' to refer to the research participant. Also, they often use a third person's views on the issue and research. In the discussion part, positivists make use of the statistical results in the data analysis and draw comments and statements.

Methodology

Methodology refers to the process and procedures of the research. It can be addressed by the question: what is the process for the research? It is the nature of research design and method. The positivists apply the scientific approach consisting of systematic and orderly procedures for researchers to study the phenomena and relationships among them (Pilot & Beck, 2004). From Smith (2006), a quasi-experimental study of quantitative research was applied as the method. The tooling including the IBS-QoL questionnaire and the Hospital Anxiety and Depression Scale questionnaire were used to measure the result of HRQoL and psychological well-being of subjects, respectively. The data collected is are the scores in questionnaire, and it was analyzed by a statistical tool, the Wilconxon signed test, to compare the results before and after the treatment. The methodology is to discover and explain relationships among variables. It will lead to the composition of e universal laws that formulate the foundation for the prediction and control of phenomena (Ponterotto, 2005). Positivists rely on four methods in quantitative research; namely descriptive, correlational, experiments and quasi-experimental methods (Burns & Grove, 2005).

In short, nursing research, as it is similar to social research, is guided by the above five assumptions with a logical order. Ontologies inform methodologies as to the nature of reality, it directs what the research is going to study. Epistemologies inform methodologies about the nature of knowledge, it directs where knowledge is to be sought. According to the previous instructions, the researchers then employ axiology, rheotorical structure and methodologies, to prepare appropriate research designs, instructing them as to where to focus their research activity, and how to recognize and extract knowledge (Sarantakos, 1993; Ponterotto, 2005).

Application of Positivistic Paradigm in Research

Quantitative research can "describe, examine relationships and determine causality between factors/variables. It stresses the measurement and analysis of causal relationships between variables. Advocates of such studies claim that their work is done from within a value-free framework" (Denzin & Lincoln, 2003, p.13). Truth in positivist research is obtained from the verification and replication of observable findings concerning directly perceivable entities or process (Poole & Jones 1996). It is useful to provide a stronger scientific base to nursing discipline for the professional development. It helps to develop knowledge and theories for improving the practice in nursing care.

According to Pilot and Beck (2004), positivist researchers apply the scientific method in quantitative research to acquire knowledge. The method consists of four characteristics: systematic/order, control, empiricism/empirical evidence, generalizability. Quantitative researchers use deductive reasoning to generate hypotheseis that are tested in the real world. They typically move in an orderly and systematic manner from identifying the research question, selection of focus, design of study in data collection and analysis methodology, to the solution of the problem. Those actions are planned in a logical series of steps by investigators. Secondly, control can help to rule out the coexisting factor that may affect the result of the study so as to increase the validity of the study. Moreover, quantitative researchers obtain empirical evidence, which is observable and sensible information, in data collection as positivism focuses on objective reality. Following the systematic and logical plan, information obtained is in numerical measurement and will be followed by statistical procedures. One of the goals of traditional scientific research is to recognize phenomena in a general approach rather than in individual cases. Therefore, the degree of generalization is an index for assessing the quality of the research. It can be optimized by matching the sampling method and sample sizes.

Limitation of Positivistic Paradigm

Traditional positivistic paradigm emphasizes s on the objectivism and view that that science that is value- free. However in the real situation, it cannot be fully value- free fully as well as objective because the values and background of the researchers affect the research to in some extentd (Holloway & Wheeler, 2010). Research can become value laden due to a variety of factors that include subjectivity and researcher bias. As so, there are scholars that realized that the reality can never be fully objective, so post-positivitism is emerged. This paradig {please insert completed sentence}

Also, there seems to be no not concern about human interactions of feelings, thoughts and perceptions of people in their research – e.g. holistic care to client (Holloway & Wheeler, 2010). Furthermore, the lack of participants' perspective within the context of their lives (Holloway & Wheeler, 2010). Due to the existence of limitation in positivistic research, there are paradigm debates and a rise of naturalistic paradigms for the complementary propose (Holloway & Wheeler, 2010). Quantitative (originated from positivism) and qualitative (originated from naturalism) researches can be used together which is called triangulation.

Conclusion

Positivistic paradigm is one of the leading paradigms in nursing research. It is essential to understand the philosophical assumptions as the justification before applying the corresponding paradigm and methodology, such as like quantitative research. Quantitative research is conducted using a scientific method with four main characteristics;, namely systematic/order, control, empirical evidence and generalization. The Nursing scholars utilized nursing research based on the scientific method to increase the evidence base knowledge. . Due to the weakness in positivistic paradigm, another paradigm called naturalistic paradigm was raised. They are not in against each otherposition, but rather have a complementary relationship rather.

Author's Background

Tam Wun San, Henry, who is a year two nursing student who is studing Master of Nursing in the from The Hong Kong Polytechnic University and Hong Kong Sanatorium Hospital. (Email: 09668839g@polyu.edu.hk)

Reference

Burns, N., & Grove, S. K. (2005). *The practice of nursing research: Conduct, critique, and utilization* (5th ed.). St. Louis, Mo.: Elsevier/Saunders.

Dempsey, P. A., Dempsey, A. D., & Dempsey, P. A. (2000). *Using nursing research: Process, critical evaluation, and utilization* (5th ed.). Philadelphia, Pa.: Lippincott.

Denzin, N. K., & Lincoln, Y. S. (2000). Introduction: The discipline and practice of qualitative research. In N. K. Denzin & Y. S. Lincoln (Eds.), *Handbook of qualitative research* (2nd ed., pp. 1–28). Thousand Oaks, CA: Sage

Denzin, N. K., & Lincoln, Y. S. (2003). *The landscape of qualitative research: Theories and issues* (2nd ed.). Thousand Oaks, Calif.: Sage Publications.

Filstead, W. J. (1979). Qualitative methods: A needed perspective in evaluation research. In T. D. Cook & C. S. Reichardt (Eds.), *Qualitative and quantitative methods in evaluation research* (pp. 33–48). Beverly Hills, CA: Sage.

Holloway, I. & Wheeler, S. (2010). *Qualitative research in nursing and healthcare (3rd ed.)*. Chichester, West Sussex, U.K.; Ames, Iowa: Wiley- Blackwell.

Linoln, Y. S., & Guba, E. G. (1985). *Naturalistic inquiry*. Beverly Hills, CA: Sage.

Polit, D. F., & Beck, C. T. (2004). *Nursing research: Principles and methods* (7th ed.). Philadelphia: Lippincott Williams & Wilkins

Polit, D. F., & Beck, C. T. (2008). *Nursing research :Generating and assessing evidence for nursing practice* (8th ed.). Philadelphia: Wolters Kluwer Health/Lippincott Williams & Wilkins.

Ponterotto, J. G. (2005). Qualitative research in counseling psychology: A primer on research paradigms and philosophy of science. *Journal of Counseling Psychology, Electronic Resource Electronic Resource, 52*(2), 126-136.

Poole, K. & Jones, A. (1996). A re-examination of the experimental design for nursing research. *Journal of Advanced Nursing.* 24, 103-114.

Powers, B. & Knapp, T. (2006). *A dictionary of nursing theory and research* (3rd ed.) Thousand Oaks, CA: Sage.

Risjord, M. W. (2010). *Nursing knowledge :Science, practice, and philosophy*. Chichester, West Sussex; Ames, Iowa: Wiley-Blackwell Pub.

Sarantakos, S. (2005). *Social research*. Basingstoke: Palgrave Macmillan.

Smith, G. D. (2006). Effect of nurse-led gut-directed hypnotherapy upon health-related quality of life in patients with irritable bowel syndrome. *Journal of Clinical Nursing, Electronic Resource Electronic Resource*, 15(6), 678-684.

Weaver, K., & Olson, J. K. (2006). *Understanding paradigms used for nursing research.* Blackwell Science Ltd.

In: Nursing Research: A Chinese Perspective
Editor: Zenobia C. Y. Chan

ISBN: 978-1-61209-833-3
©2011 Nova Science Publishers, Inc.

Chapter IV

Naturalistic Paradigm in Nursing Research

Mandy W. M. Lam and Zenobia C. Y. Chan
The Hong Kong Polytechnic University, China

Summary

"Naturalistic Paradigm" is a conceptual framework to govern the implementation of qualitative research which believes in the complexity of humans. This chapter is a review of the naturalistic paradigm, from historical review to nursing research. Applying "Naturalistic Paradigm" in nursing research, the researcher acts as an instrument, to get a rich and thick description under a natural setting as possible. It allows the researcher to understand the attached meaning of phenomenon and explore more possible associations of it, in instead of verifying a particular hypothesis. As it strongly emphasizes the presence of change, new knowledge and explanation can be generated, and considered useful to improve patient care. In this chapter, the historical review of paradigm shift and characteristics of naturalistic paradigm will be identified first identified. Then, the brief comparison of positivistic and naturalistic paradigm will be discussed. Lastly, the application of naturalistic paradigm in nursing research and its strengths and limitations will be considered.

Introduction

"Paradigm" refers a conceptual framework, underlying assumptions and perspective of studies or researches. Patton (1990) suggested that paradigm is a world view, a general perspective, a way of breaking down the complexity of the real world. While Guba (1990) stated that paradigm is an interpretative framework which is guided by a set of beliefs and perceptions about the world.

"Paradigm" constitutes both its strengths and weaknesses. As Patton (1978) suggested, that "paradigm is not only makes action possible, its weakness in that the very reason for action is hidden in the unquestioned assumption of the paradigm" (p.203).

In other words, "paradigm" is a critical component of research as it can govern the implementation of research, decides the nature and structure of questions, methods of data collection and analysis, even determines the results we get. Hence, this essay examines the shift of paradigm, overview of naturalistic paradigm and discusses the strengths and limitations of its application in nursing research.

Historical Review of Paradigm Shift

The historical development of paradigm can simply divide into three eras, including: pre-positivist, positivist and naturalist. As Wolf (1981) stated, the pre-positivist era is ranges from the time of Aristotle to 1711. During that period, Aristotle suggested two principles which are "Law of Contradiction" and "Law of Excluded Middle". Both of them are aimed to point out that there is no pro-position that can be both true and false at the same time, it must be either true or false (Mitroff and Kilmann, 1978). As Aristotle strongly believed that the world is pre-determined by god and natural motion, so all scientists should keep passive and do no harm to nature al.

However, once the scientists carry out the study, they become "active observers" doubtlessly and this change leads to the shift of paradigm, called "Positivism". "Positivism" defined as "extremely positive evaluation of science and scientific method"(Reese, 1980, p.450). Since it provides a "new rationale for the doing of science", so it causes a major impact on scientific methods rather than religious or philosophy (Lincoln and Guba, 1985, p.19). Positivists strongly believe that the world is governed by a universal law, so only the objective, controllable experiment or measurement can assist them to find out the rule and predict what happens in the future.

As Lincoln and Guba (1985) reviewed that "Positivism" was extremely and overly dependent on operationlism, it lead them ignore the meanings and implication of reality. In order to facilitate their study, most of the positivists tend to break down the subject into tiny pieces and study them in an easier way by using value-free numerical data. This technique reflects that they fail to differentiate human science and natural science. Actually, there were still different kinds of critiques about "Positivism" during that period. Some of the scholars think that positivism totally ignores the uniqueness of humans and is quite superficial sometimes (Lincoln and Guba, 1985). All of these inadequacies call for the need of changes and pass into "naturalistic paradigm". It allows the researcher to take a deeper look into of human's experience and phenomenon via naturalistic inquiry instead of using a value-free method. As it provides a new insight for analyzing a whole phenomenon, so it may useful for the improvement of the competent of care in the nursing field.

Overview of Naturalistic Paradigm

Naturalistic studies are designed to explain and understand phenomena entirely under a natural setting. Avoiding the constraint of hypothesis verification, it tries to describe the characteristics of phenomena or even explore the association among the possible variables in both micro and macro levels.

As Lincoln and Guba (1985) explained, that the characteristics of naturalistic approach will be assumed to apply in reality by using qualitative research as they possess similar principles. Firstly, qualitative research is carried y out under a "real world" setting, seeks illumination and understanding about a particular phenomenon by using in-depth interviews, observations or participant observations, . Aand the main point is the qualitative researcher concerns themselves with the importance of the meaning attached to the whole phenomenon rather than figure out the facts only. As we known, humans are constantly keep on changing, so multi- reality is always present. In other words, interesting and valuable findings and associations may originate anytime under a natural setting.

Characteristics of Naturalistic Paradigm

After we get the generally idea of naturalistic paradigm, then we can discuss some characteristics of operational naturalistic paradigm more specifically.

Firstly, the setting of naturalistic inquiry should be natural as naturalists believe that realities are whole, which cannot be measured in tiny pieces (Kuzel, 1998). A Rreality setting is the best way for them to generate ing meaning in different aspects of daily life, not only from their verbal response, but also from their daily activities or interactions with other people surrounding them.

Using the researcher as the instrument in research is a typical characteristic of naturalistic paradigm. Naturalists believe that only humans have the ability to evaluate and understand the "meaning" attach to the datan. Ccollecting and grasping information from an informant and giving an e appropriate response, such as follow up questions, in order to get more raw information as they can (Lincoln and Guba, 1985). Take in-depth interviews as example, the interview usually lasts for 1 or 2 hours and all dialogues will be analyzed by the interviewer during and after the interview. After the interview, they will transcript the dialogues and report in narrative or case study form instead of numerical data. Certainly, the information naturalists get is very rich and productive enough which may allow transferability afterward.

As qQualitative research allows and even welcomes the presence of change. Hence, researchers will not start with a complete design;, the continuing refinement and interactive process provides a chance for the researcher to explore a more and complete understanding of the subject they study. As Lincoln and Guba (1985) quoted, that the data obtained is dependent upon the quality of interaction between knower and known, so the outcome of research cannot be expected or predicted ct before the research.

Comparison of Positivistic and Naturalistic Paradigm

Here we have discussed the characteristics of natural paradigm. However, the emerging of this paradigm is not represented. The old positivistic one was being replaced as it is still widely used in nursing research nowadays. Researchers will choose the suitable one based on the purpose and of research and their owns characteristics, strengths and limitations (Lincoln and Guba, 1985). Table 1, as follows, provides a brief summary of different characteristics of positivistic and naturalistic paradigm.

Table 1. Differences between positivistic and naturalistic paradigm

Feature	Positivist Paradigm	Naturalistic Paradigm
Nature of reality	Single , tangible and fragmentable	Multiple, constructed and holistic
Relationship of knower woner to known	Independent and dualism	Interactive and inseparable
Possibility of generalization	Time and context free generalizations are possible	Only time- and context- bound working hypotheseis are possible
Possibility of causal linkages	Real cause-effect relationship	Impossible to identify cause from effects
Role of value	Value- free	Value-bound
View of truth	Confirmable	Ineluctable

Source: (Lincoln and Guba, 1985)

For people who believe in naturalistic paradigm, they do not assume that there is a single unitary reality. Since they believe that each of us is unique, so the past experiences and point of views of individuals will affect their perceptions on the same phenomena. Moreover, naturalists also believe that "knowledge is purposefully constructed" so the meaning attached to the experience is the product of social conditioning rather than individual determinationed (Lythcott & Duschl, 1990). In To contrast, the positivist holds that reality is single, testable and can be generalized. Under the "objective" and controllable experiment, they can separate themselves from the world they study and break down the complexes in different pieces and measure them one by one. Once they figure out the casual relationship between the variables, then they can control and predict the future and world directly.

Secondly, as naturalists think that the view in the context of phenomenon is the best way for understanding the reality, so they tend to keep interacting with the subject, in order to experience more. Naturalistic paradigm allows the dynamic and flexibility of research, face to face encounters between the researcher and informants directed toward understanding the informant's perspective on their lives experience as expressed in their own words. Wwhereas, positivists suggest only value- free data can maintain the neutral and "objectivity" of results, any value added into the research will be treated as "experimental errors" and are not allowed.

On the other hand, values and meaning seems as important components for naturalistic paradigm, as naturalists believe both of these can reflect the norm, culture, ideology of the society or world (Lofland & Lofland, 1996). As naturalists are more flexible to refine their questions and methods according to informant's response, so every word the researcher and informant give are important for research. This interaction is not only providing a new insight of phenomenon, it is even useful for the generation of e a new theory. As mentioned before, positivist views values and changes as "errors", which may damage the whole research, so only value- free and numerical data are valuable and favorable for them to test the hypothesis which they form prior to i the research.

In fact, the comparison between these two paradigms is not a new issue. Many scholars from different disciplines address and argue on this in the past, but have seen seem no "winner" in this battle until now. Actually, the selection of paradigm is highly depending on the aim or function of the research, no one is superior to other one inherently.

Application of Naturalistic Paradigm in Nursing Research

In the past, many worldwide universities tend to combine medical and nursing under the same school and share the same academic resources. The close relationship of the two disciplines lead scholars of nursing to adopted traditional scientific approaches easily without questioning and this restricted the development of research in the nursing field until now. Moreover, Oilver (1982) also pointed out that health research has been dominated by medical researchers which mainly used ing traditional scientific methods of positivism to test hypotheseis. Hence, it is hard to convince researchers to accept the qualitative methods which are used to generate a new hypothesis instead of verifying.

Leononger (1985) further elaborated that nurse students only learn statistical techniques in school as most of the nurse educators have been strongly socialized to use the quantitative method. In other words, they believe that it has greater validity and reliability, so they only put this paradigm in undergraduate nursing curricula,. Iignoring the importance of naturalistic paradigm because they think it is unscientific, overly subjective and biased. At the end, all nursing students only know or are keen on quantitative methods and pass it to the next generation.

Even though the publication of qualitative papers is increasing nowadays, it still stands far away from those quantitative. Then what is the advantage and importance of applying naturalistic paradigm in the clinical setting? Gorenberg (1983) mentioned that qualitative research can provide fresh insight and capture the individual's interpretation of experience via studying the individual's own lived experience directly. Wwhereas positivism only aims to find out the relationship, fail to provide the whole picture and view of the complexity and meaning of human experience, behavior and health-illness continuum, easy to miss out on the possible variables in several dimensions (Lincoln and Guba, 1985).

Nursing is not an independent profession, it is all about people, so we cannot omit the change of human beings and predict their behavior in based on "singular truth". Recently, holistic and patient- centered care has become the principle of competent care in nursing, iIf we want to provide all- around care to patient, then we should know more about their activities, perception and view of life , not just focus on numerical data. Take participate observation as an example, once the nurse researcher engaged in the clinical setting (natural setting), they will act as practitioner and nurse at the same time,. P participating in the act of "being with" the informant in their lives. Face to face interaction allows the nurse to take a deeper understanding of patients' words, activities and the meaning attached to these. That's means naturalistic research offers a well- founded approach to the study of clinical process and improve the quality of care.

It is not doubtful that quantitative method has its own effectiveness or importance as some of the data should be collected in numerical form which is easier to analyze sis and do comparison, for example: using Likert scale to measure the satisfactory level. However, the socio- cultural aspect of patients is also a need to be concerned with, and it is difficult to measure by number sometimes. Likert scale is popular in quantitative research, but the number in and of themselves can't be interpreted without understanding the assumptions which underline them,. Ttaking for example: if a researcher wants to ask the effectiveness of the treatment. The instruction shows that 1 is strongly disagree and 5 is strongly agree, then how do the respondent interpret the value "5" here? People can't really understand this quantitative value unless we dig into some of the judgments and assumptions that underlie. In fact, all knowledge is being socially constructed by socialization, cultural context. Therefore, different people may have a different understanding of the word which stated in the questionnaire, oOnly face to face interaction allows the researcher to clarify and gain more information as well.

It is clear that the function of quantitative research is used to accept or reject the hypothesis they pre-determined before the investigation. ToIn contrast, qualitative research is used to explore, discover and describe the possible new relationship with a holistic and humanistic picture via reproductive methods. Then, why is understanding the socio-cultural aspect of patients is significant for nursing research?

Research by Levins and Lewontin (1985) figured out that people tend to ignore the contribution of poverty and poor health care on tuberculosis bacillus, because they only do experiments on analyzing, testing the bacteria and measure the physiological change of the patient. They are unable to find out that the illness can be the product or problem of social, economic and class dynamic, not just a medical problem.

Moreover, unwanted pregnancy is also a complicated issue as it involves multi tli-factors in micro and macro levels, such as herself and the influence from her parents, her boyfriend and her peers. For the macro level, unwanted pregnancy can be a product of racism, inequality, context of her socio-economic class. If the researcher only uses the quantitative method to measure and focus on the teenagers' knowledge of contraception, then the data they collected will be narrow and only useful to conform to their own prediction of causal relation between the two variables (Heineman, 1994).

The Aabove studies (Levins & Lewontin, 1985; Heineman, 1994) proved that illness is not just a medical problem or singular causal relationship which can be examined by number only. It is also a social context which can only discover, reveal, explore from qualitative method, such as participate observation (PO). Through PO, we can get rich information from observation and patient's sharing which the researcher cannot predict and expect before. As people have the ability and freedom to choose the meaning of their actions, so PO allows nurse researchers to ensure whether patient's words is match with their behavior and even find out the underlying meaning behind it. Getting a new insight of the complex issue and generatinge a new idea which can also facilitate the positivist to hold a quantitative research to test the causal relationship if needed.

Limitations of Naturalistic Paradigm in Nursing Research

Although there are many advantages of naturalistic paradigm, it still has its own limitations, for example: subjectivity, ethical problems, time and expense. "Engage in meaning making together" is the feature of naturalistic paradigm, so it requires the effort and quality of both the researcher and informant. In other words, the past experience and perception of the researcher may affect the data analyzing process and even the whole research, and this "subjectivity" may lead to an incredibility of data (Krauss, 2005). Keeping the thick transcript and inter-checking with peers or supervisors can ensure the transcripts are fully explained, enhancing the trustworthiness, rigor and eliminating the bias.

Some people may worry about the ethical issue of participant observation (Heineman, 1994). However, as the researcher acts as practitioner at the same time and will not take any notes or video, so the interference of treatment or nursing care is not the main concern compared with the non-participant observation. Certainly, asking for approval, respecting the patient, building a trustful relationship and keeping confidentiality are always important for all research.

Besides, using humans as instruments and long engagements will increase the expense of research. In order to ensure the richness and usefulness of the data, several skills development of the researcher is required. Therefore, this method is better to conduct by experienced researchers rather than novice ones. Besides, it requires a long period of time to transcript, organize and analyze sis data,so all of these may lead the research cost in a more expensive way.

It is quite challenging for nursing researchers to carry out participate observations in clinical settings, as they may encounter different problems that they never think of before, therefore, and affecting the accuracy . Therefore, an audit trail,and keeping up on self-reflection are key and may help sometime.

Conclusion

Due to the functions, limitations and characteristics of positivistic and naturalistic paradigm are different, it is hard to say which paradigm is intrinsically superior to the other another one to get at truth, it is just favored by different researchers at different times with different aims. There It is no doubt that it is quite difficult for the nurse researchers using naturalistic paradigm in nursing research as it is quite a time- consuming, complex. I still believe that naturalistic paradigm positively impacts on the nursing profession in many ways as it allows new insight to emerge in different aspects. As mentioned before, illness is not just a medical problem, it can be the result of social, economic and class dynamic. Hence, a complete understanding of the patient's background and meaning of the patient's behavior is significant to improve the quality and effectiveness of nursing care delivery to the patient, especially for those sensitive or having behavioral problems.

Author's Background

Lam Wing Man, Mandy, degree of sociology, Master student of Department of Nursing at The Hong Kong Polytechnic University. (Email : mandylam_518@yahoo.com.hk)

References

Carr, L.T. (1994). The strengths and weaknesses of quantitative and qualitative research: What method for nursing? *Journal of Advanced Nursing, 20*(4), 716-721.

Glensne, C., Peshkin, P. (1992). *Becoming qualitative researches: An introduction.* New York, NY: Longman.

Golafshani, N. (2003). Understanding Reliability and Validity in Qualitative Research. *The Qualitative Report, 8*(4), 597-607.

Gorenberg, B.E. (1983). The research tradition of nursing: an emerging issue. *Nursing Research, 32*(4), 347-349.

Greene, J.C. (2008). In Tribute to Egon Guba. *Qualitative Injuiry, 14*(8), 1360-1365.

Heineman Pieper, M. (1994). *Science, not scientism: The robustness of naturalistic clinical research.* In E. Sherman & W. Reid. (Eds.), Qualitative research in social work (pp. 71-88). New York, NY: Columbia.

Krauss, S.E. (2005). Research Paradigms and Meaning Maker: A Primer. *The Qualitative Report, 10*(4), 758-770.

Kuzel, A.J. (1998). Naturalistic Inquiry: An Appropriate Model for Family Medicine. *Special Series el : Classics From Family Medicine, 30*(9), 665-671.

Leininger, M.M. (Ed.). (1985). *Qualitative research method in nursing.* Orlando, FL: Grune & Stratton.

Levins, R., Lewontin, R.C. (1985). *The Dialectical Biologist.* Cambridge: Harvard University Press.

Lincoln, Y.S., Guba, E.G. (1985). *Naturalistic inquiry.* Beverly Hills, CA:Sage.

Lincoln, Y.S., Guba, E.G. (2000). Paradigmatic controversies, contradictions and emerging confluences. In N. K. Denzin & Y. S. Lincoln (Eds.), *Handbook of Qualitative Research* (2nd ed., pp. 163-188). Thousand Oaks, CA: Sage Publications, Inc.

Lofland, J., Lofland, L. (1996). *Analyzing social setting* (3rd ed.) Belmont, CA: Wadsworth.

Lythcott, J., Duschl, R. (1990). Qualitative research: From methods to conclusion. *Science Education, 74* (4), 449-460.

Merriam, S.B., Heuer, B. (1996). Meaning-making, adult learning and development: A model with implications for practice. *International Journal of Lifelong Education, 15*(4), 243-255.

Mitroff, I. I., Kilmann, R. H. (1978). *Methodlogical approaches to social science.* San Francisco: Jossey-Bass.

Morgan, A. K., Drury, V. B. (2003). Legitimizing the Subjectivity of Human Reality Through Qualitative Research Method. *The Qualitative Report, 8*(1), 70-80.

Morse, J.M., Field, P. A. (1995). *Qualitative research methods for health professionals* (2nd ed.). Thousand Oaks, CA: Sage.

Oilver, C. J. (1982). The phenomenological approach in nursing research. *Nursing Research*, *31*(3), 178-181.

Patton, M.Q. (1978). *Utilization-focused evaluation.* Beverly Hills, CA: Sage.

Patton, M.Q. (1990). *Qualitative Evaluation and Research Methods* (2nd ed.). Newbury Park, CA: Sage.

Pullen, M. (2000). Understanding research paradigms in nursing research. *ADF Health*, *1*(1), 124-128.

Reese, W. L. (1980). *Dictionary of philosophy and religious.* Atlantic Highlands, NJ: Humanities.

Seale, C. (1999). Quality in qualitative research. *Qualitative Inquiry, 5*(4), 465-478.

Wolf, F. A. (1981). *Taking the quantum leap.* San Franciso: Harper & Row.

In: Nursing Research: A Chinese Perspective
Editor: Zenobia C. Y. Chan

ISBN: 978-1-61209-833-3
©2011 Nova Science Publishers, Inc.

Chapter V

Naturalistic Paradigm

Lina T. W. Wong and Zenobia C. Y. Chan
The Hong Kong Polytechnic University, China

Summary

This essay is an overview of naturalistic paradigm. The aim of this essay is to obtain an understanding of naturalistic paradigm, from philosophical aspects to its application on research studies. Paradigm is a set of philosophical beliefs on ontology, epistemology and methodology aspects. For naturalistic paradigm, on the ontological aspect, it believes that reality is multiple and subjectively constructed. On the epistemological aspect, it believes that knowledge is created and obtained from an interactive process. On the methodology aspect, it usually associates with qualitative method which emphasizes on collecting narrative information. Naturalistic paradigm emerged from critique toward the traditional research paradigm, positivist paradigm. Therefore, it is a contradicting paradigm towards positivism. Naturalistic and positivist paradigm are two major research paradigms which are often associated with qualitative and quantitative studies, respectively. By contrasting, these two paradigms, it identifies the strength of naturalistic paradigm on addressing research which is sensitive to humanness, such as anthropological and sociological studies. Naturalistic paradigm can be applied y on research studies, from formulating queries y to reporting research findings. Therefore, it is important to understand research paradigm before conducting research.

Introduction

Nowadays, more researches are turning away from the dominant quantitative study and conducting researches through qualitative study (Agostinho, 2005; Barrington, 1994; Luczun, 1990; Mulhall & Jones, 1995; Sogoric, Middleton, Lang, Ivankovic, & Kern, 2005; Williams, 2005). Researchers are now paying more attention to qualitative study and therefore, leading to the expanding of multiple research designs (e.g. ethnography, phenomenology) and methods (e.g. interview, focus group, participatory) (S. N. Hesse-Biber & Leavy, 2006). What leads to the increasing awareness on qualitative study? In fact, actions are always guided by the underlining belief. Previously, the positivism paradigm, which has a close association with quantitative study, is the dominant belief on research (DePoy & Gitlin, 1994). However, researchers started to criticize the idea of objectivity and single reality of traditional beliefs and it leads to the emerging of a new paradigm, the naturalistic paradigm (Lincoln & Guba, 1985). This new paradigm indicates a new page on research. As the flexible design of qualitative study can fit into the philosophical belief of naturalist paradigm on the nature of reality (ontology), the nature of knowledge (epistemology), and the methods to obtain knowledge (methodology), emerge of naturalistic paradigm contributing e to the expanding of qualitative study (S. N. Hesse-Biber & Leavy, 2006).

Though today researchers today are more aware of the importance of qualitative research, many researchers ignore the underlining naturalistic paradigm and philosophical belief (Denzin & Lincoln, 2000). It is because when qualitative research is established well in the framework of naturalistic paradigm, it facilitates researchers to carry out research without going through a long philosophical consideration on ontology, epistemology and methodology (Lincoln & Guba, 1985). However, the paradigm also hides itself behind the title of qualitative research (Denzin & Lincoln, 2000). Therefore, the paradigm becomes invisible to many researchers (Denzin & Lincoln, 2000).

As a researcher, it is important to understand naturalistic paradigm which indicates an important change on research design and methodology. Understanding naturalistic paradigm can help researchers to obtain a more in-depth understanding and justification on the choice of method, setting and analysis of qualitative study (Erlandson, 1993; Guba, 1978; Lincoln & Guba, 1985; Miller & Fredericks, 2002). Also, it can prepare researchers to understand the philosophical aspect on emerging paradigms following the naturalistic paradigm (Denzin & Lincoln, 2000). The development of a research paradigm is on an emancipating stage in which the belief of naturalistic paradigm may reformulate and new paradigms are emerging (Denzin & Lincoln, 2000).

The objective of this essay is underpinning the importance to understand naturalistic paradigm in order to obtain a more holistic understanding towards research design and methodology. This essay is consists ed of (a) an introduction of naturalistic paradigm through the transition from positivism to naturalism, followed by with (b) the comparison between naturalistic and positivist paradigm and then (c) the application of naturalistic paradigm in research.

Research Paradigm

Before introducing naturalistic paradigm, it is necessary to clarify the meaning of research paradigm. Paradigm is a set of basic beliefs or world view on three main aspects which are ontology, epistemology and methodology (Doordan, 1998; S. N. Hesse-Biber & Leavy, 2006). In which, oOntology refers to study of the nature of reality, for example reality is single or multiple, objective or subject (DePoy & Gitlin, 1994; Lincoln & Guba, 1985). Epistemology refers to the theory of knowledge which concerns ing the way knowledge is created, validity of knowledge and also the relationship between the researcher and research participant, for example whether the researcher is independent or interacts with the participant (DePoy & Gitlin, 1994; Doordan, 1998). Methodology refers to the method used to obtain knowledge, for example; experimental, hermeneutical and dialectical methods (DePoy & Gitlin, 1994; Doordan, 1998). These set of beliefs are said to be basic because the ultimate truthfulness of these philosophical beliefs cannot be proven, people can only accept them on faith (Lincoln & Guba, 1985). Therefore, they are also referred to as assumptions of the paradigm (Polit & Beck, 2006). These basic beliefs can act as a framework for research or theories construction (S. N. Hesse-Biber & Leavy, 2006). Then it can help to shape research designs and method (S. N. Hesse-Biber & Leavy, 2006). However, it also influences researcher's perspectives or world views. Therefore, Guba & Lincoin (1985) suggested that "while paradigms are thus enabling, they are also constraining".

Positivism to Naturalistic Paradigm

As paradigm or world view is often affected by the social condition which is continuously changing in human history, there is no single universal paradigm (Denzin & Lincoln, 2000; Lincoln & Guba, 1985). As mentioned before in the history of research, there is a major shift of paradigm from the dominant positivism to naturalistic paradigm (Guba, 1978; Lincoln & Guba, 1985). In order to understand naturalistic paradigm, it is essential to know why new paradigm is needed (Lincoln & Guba, 1985). Naturalistic paradigm arises due to the disagreement of people towards the basic belief of positivism (Erlandson, 1993). It is then constructed based on the critique on positivism (Lincoln & Guba, 1985). Therefore, contrasting the differences between positivism and naturalistic paradigm on philosophical beliefs including ontological, epistemological and methodological aspects can reveal not only the weakness of positivism but. I it also reflects the strength of naturalistic paradigm on conducting research.

Ontological Beliefs

On the ontological aspect, positivism believes that there is "real" and single reality which is only objectively affected by natural causes (Denzin & Lincoln, 2000; Doordan, 1998). It ignores human nature that all people perceive the world differently (Lincoln & Guba, 1985),. Wwhile naturalistic paradigm believes that there are "relative" and multiple realities which are subjectively constructed by individuals (Denzin & Lincoln, 2000; Doordan, 1998). It is because people always perceive the world in different ways and perception can change over time and different locations (Lincoln & Guba, 1985).

Epistemological Beliefs

On the epistemological aspect, positivism believes that researchers are finding the objective reality (Doordan, 1998; Polit & Beck, 2006). Also, researchers and samples are independent from each other (Denzin & Lincoln, 2000). Therefore, researchers can investigate the samples objectively without influencing the participants or being influenced (Denzin & Lincoln, 2000). This belief assumes that the sample can be strictly controlled and any influence can be eliminated (DePoy & Gitlin, 1994). However, if the sample is not an object but a human, it is difficult to impose strict control as it may be unethical (DePoy & Gitlin, 1994), . Wwhile naturalistic paradigm believes that researchers are finding that it is the subjective reality created during the interaction between researcher and participant (Polit & Beck, 2006).

Methodological Beliefs

On the methodological aspect, positivism usually adopts the experimental and manipulative methods in which variables can be better controlled and subjectivity can be limited by using quantitative study with measurable data (Doordan, 1998; Polit & Beck, 2006). This methodological approach ignores the humanness, for example, the study on human experience and feelings cannot be quantified (Lincoln & Guba, 1985). Also, it can be unethical to impose control and manipulation on human subjects (DePoy & Gitlin, 1994),. Wwhile naturalistic paradigm adopts the hermeneutical and dialectical methods, in which the findings are obtained through the interaction between researchers and participants (Denzin & Lincoln, 2000). The subjective and multiple realities can be studied through qualitative study by the gathering of context-based or narrative data (Doordan, 1998). This methodological approach takes humanness into account, for example, it allows the study of human experiments and feelings (Lincoln & Guba, 1985).

Based on the comparison, it reveals that the major difference between paradigms is whether humanness is taken into account or not (Lincoln & Guba, 1985). For naturalistic paradigm, the humanness is always involved in the consideration of the nature of reality and knowledge. This implies that naturalistic paradigm is especially important for research that is sensitive to humanness, such as anthropological and sociological studies (Athen, 2010; DePoy & Gitlin, 1994; Polit & Beck, 2006). It reflects the strength of applying naturalistic paradigm on human-related research. Apart from this, it is important to note that differences between the two paradigms are so large that some beliefs are even contradicted, for example, one is seeking the objective real and the other is seeking relative real which is subjective (Denzin & Lincoln, 2000; Lincoln & Guba, 1985). Therefore, they are incommensurable and naturalistic paradigm denotes a major shift of research paradigm throughout the history of research (Lincoln & Guba, 1985).

Application of Naturalistic Paradigm

This major shift of belief towards the naturalistic view on reality and knowledge has initiated a great change on how researchers perform their studies (S. N. Hesse-Biber & Leavy, 2006). When applying naturalistic paradigm on research, there are at least three major ideas we have to bear in mind. Firstly, we have to believe that realities are multiple and subjectively constructed (Lincoln & Guba, 1985). Secondly, knowledge can be obtained through human-to-human interaction (Lincoln & Guba, 1985). Thirdly, the most important is keeping a high awareness on humanness factors because the philosophical beliefs of naturalistic paradigm in fact, rise from the increasing awareness of humanness in the society (Lincoln & Guba, 1985). These three ideas are an important guide on each research stage mentioned below, from formulating research queries to reporting the findings.

Formulating Research Queries

The first stage of research is to formulate research queries. Research query is a question that the researcher wants to answer by conducting the research (DePoy & Gitlin, 1994). Naturalistic study usually adopts a broad query at the beginning (DePoy & Gitlin, 1994). The intention is based on the belief that multiple realities exist and the query should be broad enough to obtain the multiple realities (Erlandson, 1993). After data collection and analysis, the multiple realities can be revealed from the broad query (Erlandson, 1993). Then, researchers may re-formulate the query into more specific questions which they are interested in for further, in-depth study (DePoy & Gitlin, 1994). For the theme of query, it depends on the type of research designs being chosen. If it is ethnography, the query focuses on the concern of cultural meaning or patterns of certain groups (Doordan, 1998). If it is phenomenology, the query focuses concern of human experience on certain situations (Doordan, 1998).

Choosing Research Design

The second stage of research is choosing a research design. Research design is an overall plan for conducting research and addressing the query, from formulating research queries to reporting the finding (DePoy & Gitlin, 1994). Naturalistic studies usually adopt flexible research designs in which the design is not fixed before the start of research (Erlandson, 1993). In fact, the research design is often revised throughout naturalistic study (DePoy & Gitlin, 1994). This is based on the belief that knowledge is obtained though human interaction (Polit & Beck, 2006). Therefore, the research study is not only guided by the researchers, it can also be influenced by the participants (Erlandson, 1993). Throughout the interaction between researchers and participants, researchers may adjust the research design to match the changing or emerging focus (DePoy & Gitlin, 1994). Apart from being flexible, qualitative design is a common feature of different naturalistic research designs. In which, context-based or narrative data is collected instead of measurable quantitative data (Doordan, 1998). It is because naturalistic knowledge is generated through human interaction which cannot be quantified or represented with numerical value (Polit & Beck, 2006). For example, there are different types of naturalistic research designs, such as ethnography, phenomenology and grounded theory (DePoy & Gitlin, 1994). Different types of research designs can be chosen based on the different focuses of the study, for example, grounded theory for generating theory and phenomenology for discovering the meaning of lived experience (DePoy & Gitlin, 1994). However, it is common that the data collected is context-based or narrative, such as an interview strip, field notes and audio-tape (Marshall & Rossman, 2006; Mulhall, 2003).

Defining Setting and Boundary

The third stage of research is defining as setting and boundary. Setting refers to the physical location or environment in where the information is gathered (DePoy & Gitlin, 1994). A Nnaturalistic study should be conducted in a natural setting which refers to gathering research information in a setting that participants are commonly found, such as home and the working place (Doordan, 1998; Lincoln & Guba, 1985). It is because based on the naturalistic beliefs; multiple realities can only be understood as a whole and in a holistic manner (Lincoln & Guba, 1985). Therefore, naturalistic realities should not be studied in a fragmented manner as positivism (Lincoln & Guba, 1985). For positivism in an experimental setting, except for the dependent and independent variables being studied, other variables are strictly controlled (DePoy & Gitlin, 1994). This kind of study only reveals realities in one dimension which is the relationship between dependent and independent variables (DePoy & Gitlin, 1994). This neglects the complex condition in a natural situation and masks the possibility of multiple realities (Lincoln & Guba, 1985). In contrast, a natural setting reveals complex and multiple realities in a real situation (Erlandson, 1993). Boundary refers the limits being set on the type of concept explored, participant involved and information gathered (DePoy & Gitlin, 1994). For the sampling boundary of naturalistic study, it mainly adopts purposive sampling (Erlandson, 1993; Lincoln & Guba, 1985). In purposive sampling, participants of the naturalistic study are deliberately selected based on some pre-defined criteria rather than sampling randomly (Polit & Beck, 2006). It is because random or representative sampling, which are aimed as representing the population, is likely to mask the deviant case therefore, multiple realities cannot be identified (Lincoln & Guba, 1985). While purposive sampling allows a purposive study of some minor groups or deviant cases, it can reveal the multiple realities (Lincoln & Guba, 1985). As the naturalistic sampling is aimed at ts obtaining multiple realities but not generalization, so therefore small sampling size is acceptable (Erlandson, 1993).

Gathering Information

The fourth stage of research is gathering information. Gathering information refers to the investigative action carried out by the researcher to obtain information that helps to answer the research query (DePoy & Gitlin, 1994). There are two characteristics for naturalistic information gathering. Firstly, it involves the active participation of researchers because naturalistic study is obtaining knowledge through interaction between researchers and participants (Erlandson, 1993; Lincoln & Guba, 1985). Secondly, naturalistic researchers always use multiple data-gathering methods to obtain multiple realities (DePoy & Gitlin, 1994). There are multiple data-gathering methods for naturalistic study and new data-gathering methods are continuously emerging (DePoy & Gitlin, 1994). It is because naturalistic paradigm facilitates the emergence t of new data-gathering methods. Based on naturalistic belief, knowledge is created through researcher-and-participant interaction and there are unlimited types of interaction, for example, interviews can be conducted through the interaction of asking questions, participant observation can be conducted through the interaction of researchers getting into groups and creating field notes and , focus group studies y can be conducted through discussion among participants (DePoy & Gitlin, 1994;

Polit & Beck, 2006). Therefore, there is always the emerging of new data-gathering methods for naturalistic study (Lincoln & Guba, 1985). Researchers should be open-minded to adopt new data-gathering methods, as long as narrative data is explored through human interaction.

Analysis of Data

The fifth stage is analyzing data. For naturalistic studies, inductive reasoning is suitable to identify multiple realties and obtain a general meaning from the realties (DePoy & Gitlin, 1994). Inductive reasoning refers to the human reasoning process in which general is evolved from specific, for example, general meaning of value can evolve from specific case and observation (Lincoln & Guba, 1985).

Evaluating Quality of Study

The sixth stage is evaluating the quality of study. For naturalistic studies, a specific set of criterions including credibility, transferability, dependability and conformability are required to justify the trustworthiness and quality of of thestudy (Polit & Beck, 2006; Tobin & Begley, 2004). The quality criterions for traditional positivism, including validity, reliability and generalizability, fail to apply on naturalistic paradigm (DePoy & Gitlin, 1994; Polit & Beck, 2006). It is because the nature of query and data collected are completely different between naturalistic and positivism studies.

Reporting the Findings

The seventh stage is reporting the findings. Reporting refers to the writing of reports which summarizes the research process, findings and conclusions clearly (DePoy & Gitlin, 1994). The aim of reporting is to share and disseminate the conclusion of the research. Case study reporting mode is preferred for reporting a naturalistic study. The descriptive nature of a case study report allows a clear presentation of the interaction process between researchers and participants. The interaction is the knowledge- creating process of naturalistic paradigm. Therefore, a case study report is suitable for reporting a naturalistic study. In fact, there are different formats for reporting a naturalistic study. Other reporting modes can be used if they can facilitate the reporting of detailed and descriptive information.

Based on the application, the characteristics of naturalistic studies are similar to qualitative studies (S. N. Hesse-Biber & Leavy, 2006). When applying the naturalistic paradigm, people may equalize naturalistic paradigm to qualitative studies. However, it is important to distinguish them. Naturalistic paradigm is a set of beliefs on the nature of reality and knowledge (Lincoln & Guba, 1985). It should be used consistently throughout the whole study. You cannot believe in both single and multiple realities at the same time. You can only choose to believe in either naturalistic paradigm or positivism. The two contradicting beliefs cannot exist in the same research (Lincoln & Guba, 1985). On the other hand, qualitative study mainly refers to a research method used to obtain descriptive and narrative data which are subjective in nature (Doordan, 1998). It does not contradict or exclude the use of quantitative method in the same research (Polit & Beck, 2006). A Mmixed research method is an example which adopts both qualitative and quantitative methods in a single study (S. Hesse-Biber, 2010; S. N. Hesse-Biber & Leavy, 2006). Therefore, within a single study, researchers should apply naturalistic paradigm consistently in each research stage.

Conclusion

To conclude, naturalistic paradigm is a set of beliefs or world views in which reality is seen m as multiple and subjectively constructed and knowledge can be created and obtained through human interaction (Denzin & Lincoln, 2000; Lincoln & Guba, 1985). This paradigm emerged from the critique on the traditional positivism therefore, the basic beliefs of naturalistic and positivist paradigm on ontology, epistemology and methodology are contradicting (Lincoln & Guba, 1985). By contrasting, these two paradigms, it shows the strength of naturalistic paradigm on addressing human-related research, such as anthropological and sociological studies. Research paradigm is a guide to justify the choice of a research design (Erlandson, 1993). Naturalistic paradigm is often the underlying belief to support the qualitative research design (S. N. Hesse-Biber & Leavy, 2006). Therefore, it is important to understand naturalistic paradigm before conducting qualitative research.

Author's Background

Wong Tik Wun, Lina, a year two student who is studying Master of Nursing in the Hong Kong Polytechnic University and the Hong Kong Sanatorium Hospital. (Email: linatik@hotmail.com)

References

Agostinho, S. (2005). Naturalistic inquiry in e-learning research. *International Journal of Qualitative Methods, 4*(1).

Athen, L. (2010). Naturalistic inquiry in theory and practice. *Journal of Contemporary Ethnography, 39*(1), 87-125.

Barrington, R. (1994). A naturalistic inquiry of post-operative pain after therapeutic touch. *NLN Publ*(14-2607), 199-213.

Denzin, N. K., & Lincoln, Y. S. (2000). *The handbook of qualitative research* (2nd ed.). Thousand Oaks, Calif. : Sage.

DePoy, E., & Gitlin, L. N. (1994). *Introduction to research : multiple strategies for health and human services* St. Louis: Mosby.

Doordan, A. M. (1998). *Lippincott's need-to-know : research survival guide* Philadelphia: Lippincott.

Erlandson, D. A. (1993). *Doing naturalistic inquiry : a guide to methods*. Newbury Park, Calif.: Sage.

Guba, E. G. (1978). *Toward a methodology of naturalistic inquiry in educational evaluation* Los Angeles, Calif.: Center for the Study of Evaluation, UCLA Graduate School of Education, University of California.

Hesse-Biber, S. (2010). Qualitative approaches to mixed methods practice. *Qualitative Inquiry 16*(6), 455-468.

Hesse-Biber, S. N., & Leavy, P. (2006). *The practice of qualitative research.* Thousand Oaks.: Sage Publications.

Lincoln, Y. S., & Guba, E. G. (1985). *Naturalistic inquiry*. Newbury Parks, Calif. : Sage

Luczun, M. E. (1990). Naturalistic inquiry in practice. *J Post Anesth Nurs, 5*(2), 115-116.

Marshall, C., & Rossman, G. B. (2006). *Designing qualitative research* (4th ed.). Thousands Oaks, Calif.: Sage

Miller, S. I., & Fredericks, M. (2002). Naturalistic inquiry and reliabilism: a compatible epistemological grounding. *Qual Health Res, 12*(7), 982-989.

Mulhall, A. (2003). In the field: notes on observation in qualitative research. *J Adv Nurs, 41*(3), 306-313.

Mulhall, A., & Jones, A. (1995). Medicine and nursing. Medicine and nursing need both scientific and naturalistic inquiry. *BMJ, 311*(7009), 872.

Polit, D. F., & Beck, C. T. (2006). *Essentials of nursing research : methods, appraisal, and utilization* (6th ed.). Philadelphia, PA.: Lippincott Williams & Wilkins.

Sogoric, S., Middleton, J., Lang, S., Ivankovic, D., & Kern, J. (2005). A naturalistic inquiry on the impact of interventions aiming to improve the health and the quality of life in the community. *Soc Sci Med, 60*(1), 153-164.

Tobin, G. A., & Begley, C. M. (2004). Methodological rigour within a qualitative framework. *J Adv Nurs, 48*(4), 388-396.

Williams, C. M. (2005). The identification of family members' contribution to patients' care in the intensive care unit: a naturalistic inquiry. *Nurs Crit Care, 10*(1), 6-14.

In: Nursing Research: A Chinese Perspective   ISBN: 978-1-61209-833-3
Editor: Zenobia C. Y. Chan   ©2011 Nova Science Publishers, Inc.

Chapter VI

A Guide to Answer
your Research Question

S. S. Pang and Zenobia C. Y. Chan
The Hong Kong Polytechnic University, China

Summary

Research design is the guide map for the researcher to find out the answer to the research question and it is the most important planning stage in the research process. This article focuses on the selection of the research design with examples of clinical research. Before studying various research designs, criteria of good research designs are discussed to let the novice researcher understand the elements and considerations in order to answer the research question in-depth, effectively and efficiently. Two main research design approaches, quantitative and qualitative research studies y are discussed with their strengths and limitations and implications in nursing and healthcare research.

Introduction

This article is to discuss the relationship between the question the research sets out to answer and the research design used to answer this question. In practice, the research question is the spirit in preparing the research project. So, how deep and how wide the researcher answers the research question are also the crucial factors to the quality and validity of the research project. Doubtless, research design is the map of the territory, that is to say it is a plan that governs the conduct of the research, albeit being dynamic and flexible. Factors affecting the design of the research revolve mainly around the research question and the investigators knowledge of the research topic and methodologies (Freshwater & Bishop, 2004). However, there is substantial information describing various kinds of research design but no definite guidance indicating to the researcher whether it is appropriate to use such a research design. Therefore, it is easy to confuse novice researchers because conducting a research project involves a series of steps and is time- consuming from several months to years. Research design is the guide to lead the researcher to answer the question. It is important for researcher to learn how to identify the study design so as to evaluate threats to validity results from design flaws. In addition, this article aims to assist researchers to decide which research design, qualitative or quantitative, will best answer their questions.

This article consists of two major sections. The first section will explore the term of research question and research design. An Ooverview of various types of design, their strengths and limitations are discussed with examples in nursing and healthcare studies. The second part will examine the relationship between the research question and the research design and demonstrate how the research design answers the research question appropriately.

Research Question

Research question is not only the researchable problem which allows the researcher identifying the topic of research project, but it also leads the researcher answer how wide and how deep to the research question. Cormack and Benton (1996) distinguish between two types of research question- interrogative and declarative. An interrogative research question is expressed as a question and alludes to a gap in health care knowledge. An example might be "What is the experience of older people following discharge from hospital?" A declarative question is a statement that clearly defines the purpose of the study. For example, "the purpose of this study is to examine the relationship between systematic discharge preparations and hospital readmission rates in a group of older people". Different types of research question will generate different types of knowledge. So the way in which the research question is expressed will be dependent upon whether the researcher is seeking to generate either descriptive, explanatory or predictive knowledge.

Research Design

A research design is a blueprint for conducting a study and overall plan of how the researcher intends to implement the project in practice. The purpose of a design is to maximize the possibility of obtaining valid answers to research questions or hypotheses (Parahoo, 1997). These questions can result in research driven by a researcher's curiosity or interest in a theoretical question and the goal is to improve the client's health care condition. A good design provides the subjects, the setting, and the protocol within which these comparisons can be clearly examined. Critiquing a design involves examining the study environment, sample, treatment, and measurement.

So, the research design addresses the planning of the scientific inquiry: anticipating subsequent stages of the research project, including choosing the research method; identifying the unit of analysis and the variables to be measured; establishing procedures for data collection; and devising an analysis strategy. Thinking through and planning for the critical stages of research in advance can prevent important omissions and reduce serious errors (Shi, 2008).

Quantitative Research Design

When a research question is attempting to generate explanatory or predictive knowledge, quantitative research design is the choice (Draper, 2004). The quantitative research is concerned with applying theories and techniques to assist in the manipulation of the data. The scientific method, which is the basis of quantitative research, requires that a research proposes a theory and subjects that theory to empirical testing (Berglund, 2001).

There are four types of research design commonly used in nursing and healthcare research; ch, namely, descriptive, correlational, quasi-experimental, and experimental (Burns & Grove, 2007). Descriptive and correlational studies examine variables in natural environments and do not include treatments provided by the researcher. Quasi-experimental and experimental studies are designed to examine cause and effect. In correlational designs, a large range in the variable scores is necessary to determine the existence of a relationship. Thus, the sample should reflect the full range of scores possible on the variables being measured. Experimental and comparison subjects are selected from the same pool of potential subjects. Comparison and treatment groups may evolve naturally. Experimental design is developed for a variety of studies focused on examining causality.

Qualitative Research Design

When a research question is attempting to generate exploratory or descriptive knowledge, qualitative research methods are most appropriate (Draper, 2004). Qualitative research is any kind of research that produces findings not arrived at by means of quantification (Strauss & Corbin, 1990). Themes for qualitative inquiry usually focus on an in-depth study of real world situations over time without manipulating them. Three common qualitative research approaches, namely ethnography, phenomenology and grounded theory are examined.

Ethnography is concerned with describing people in their cultural context and it has its roots in social anthropology and focuses on small scale communities traditionally (Draper 2004). For instance, Holland (1999) explored the transition from student nurse to qualified nurse using an ethnographic approach. She undertook participant observations and interviews in practice settings, along with open-ended questionnaires. Ethnography has the potential therefore, to be highly reflexive because the researcher acknowledges how their particular cultural location, values and beliefs.

Phenomenology is concerned with understanding the individual experience which emphasizes the complexity of human experience and the need to study that experience as it is actually lived (Polit & Hungler, 1991). For example, King and Turner (2000) undertook a Husserlian phenomenological study to explore the experiences of registered nurses caring for adolescent girls with anorexia in Australia. Data was ere analyzed and six themes emerged: personal core values of nurses; core values challenged; emotional turmoil; frustration; turning points; and resolution.

Grounded theory is an inductive approach to generate knowledge and theories or hypotheses emerge from or are grounded in the data (Crookes & Davies, 2004). A key difference from other qualitative methods is that researchers start their data collection and from this ese initial data, begin to formulate a theory, which is then subsequently developed and confirmed through further data collection. For example, Levy (1999) conducted a grounded theory study to investigate the processes by which midwives facilitate women to make informed choices over their pregnancy and delivery. Interactions between midwives and women were observed and interviews were also conducted with the midwives.

Sometimes it is difficult to distinguish between the three approaches and Parahoo (1997, p.46) summarizes it as below:

> Phenomenology collects data on individuals' experiences as its focus is on individuals. In ethnography, individuals are studied as part of their environment and the focus is on individuals not in isolation, but in relation to their institutions, organizations, communities, customs or policies. Both of these approaches seek mainly to describe phenomena rather than to explain them. In grounded theory, the focus is on the generation of theories from data and it therefore matters little if individuals are studied in isolation or as part of their cultural and social environment.

In summary, quantitative designs focuses on approaches that emphasize explanation of variables, verification of data, measuring variables, use of instruments for data collection, statistical significance and internal validity. Qualitative designs emphasize the understanding of social action, discovery of information, meaning of concepts, participatory involvement of researcher as a means of data collection, and trustworthiness of findings as corroborated by the participants in the research.

As quantitative design and qualitative design have their own strengths and limitations respectively, the researcher use mixed methods, like triangulation to conduct their research in order to find out the results and knowledge. For example, Weiss, Fawcett and Aber (2009) employ both qualitative and quantitative methods to study "Adaptation, postpartum concerns, and learning needs in the first two weeks after caesarean birth" which uses a mixed descriptive research design.

Relationship between Research Question and Research Design

There are three levels of questions. Level I are those questions asking "what is" or what are"; Level II are those questions asking "what is/are the relationship among variables"; Level III are those questions asking "why" and "Hhow". If the question is more outcome-oriented, it leads the researcher to a quantitative design. On the other hand, if the question is process-oriented, a qualitative design is more appropriate to the researcher.

The following table summarizes the level of research questions and suggested research designs with examples.

If the nurse researcher seeks to determine whether a new treatment for a chronic disease significantly improves outcomes over and above current "best practices", it is required to compare outcomes by using a quantitative method. If the nurse researcher seeks to determine whether application of multi-disciplinary quality improvement processes significantly increase the likelihood of better patient outcomes than a medical per review process alone, a quantitative method will determine the quantitative changes but qualitative methods will elicit barriers to implementation or incidents critical to success. If the nurse researcher seeks to understand what factors influence patients in making decisions about health care treatments, a qualitative method is required to reveal their underlying values, cognitive processes and discourse about treatment effectiveness for example (Berglund, 2001).

As mentioned previously, the quantitative research is primarily concerned with "What", "Where", and "When" of research while . And, qualitative research is concerned with the "How" and "Why" of research (Maltby, Williams, McGarry & Day, 2010). We are going to discuss how research design helps the researcher answer different levels of research question.

Table 1. The level of Research Question and Suggested Research Designs with Examples

Level	Research Question	Example	Suggested Research Design
I	What is/are?	What is the cultural practice of women in Hong Kong during the postpartum period?	Qualitative research design Advantages: This is an open- ended question and researchers can let the participant express their idea and experience freely.
II	What is the relationship among variables?	What is the relationship between socio-economic class and postpartum depression?	Quantitative research design Advantages: Researchers can identify various socio-economic classes by family income group to justify the severity of postpartum depression.
III	Why and How?	How do student nurses transit to qualified nurse after graduation?	Qualitative research design Advantages: Researchers can play the role as participant observer to explore the physical, psychological changes and transition process.

Level I Research Question

A Level I research question is looking for the fact. Therefore, a descriptive study is applicable to find out the factual information by means of qualitative research design. For example, a nurse researcher is going to study the postpartum nursing care to a new mother in Hong Kong and determines the research question as "What is the cultural practices of women in Hong Kong during the postpartum period?". By applying a qualitative research design, the researcher is able to interview women about their self- care practices within the family home during the month after the birth of their first child.

Descriptive studies are designed to gain more information about variables within a particular field of study. The descriptive study is designed to gain more information about characteristics within a particular field of study. Its purpose is to provide a picture of a situation as it naturally happens. A descriptive design may be used to develop theories, identify problems with current practice, justify a current practice, make judgments, or determine what other practitioners in similar situations are doing.

Level II Research Question

A Level II research question is to examine relationships between or among two or more variables in a single group and quantitative research design is more practical to find out the answer. For instance, a leg ulcer specialist nurse is trying to decide on the most effective methods for treating patients' leg ulcers- using a short-stretch bandage or a medium-stretch one? How would the nurse assess the effectiveness of the dressing? Through its (1) comfort, (2) ability to alleviate pain or (3) effect on how quickly the leg ulcer heals? All three ways of looking at the effectiveness of a type of dressing can be labeled "variables" as they can vary for different groups of patients and depending on how severe the leg ulcer is (another variable). Nurse researchers would apply the quasi-experimental design to control as many threats to validity as possible in a situation in which some of the components of true experimental design are lacking

Level III Research Question

A Level III research question is to explore the reason, process to explain the presence of phenonmenon. In-depth understanding and observation to the participants are useful to let the researcher explore the additional, unexpected information which would not be reflected from data collection in the quantitative research approach. For example, the nurse researcher is going to study why the teenagers abuse the drugs though they know that drug abuse is harmful to their health. If the researcher applies the qualitative research design and methodologies, like focus groups, case study and personal interviews, the reason covers holistically including their lifestyles, culture, values. Such design assists to find out how the dynamic of an experience influences subsequent behavior.

It is unfair to judge which research design and approaches are is better because they are different. Both quantitative and qualitative research designs have their strengths and limitations. However, it is important for the nurse researcher to be is able to understand and compare the characteristics, methodologies, strengths and weaknesses of various designs when selecting the appropriate design to match the study requirements and constraints.

Conclusion

The overall purpose of the research is to find an answer to the research question. An appropriate and well-executed research design ensures that this is done in the most rigorous way possible. The purpose of design is to set up a situation that maximizes the possibilities of obtaining accurate responses to objectives, questions, or hypotheses. A good design provides the subjects, the setting, and the protocol within which those comparisons can be clearly examined.

The type of research can be reflected by the methods section of a research report. Different research designs require different levels of researcher and participant relationship. If the researcher acts as an objective observer, quantitative research design is appropriate and is required to consider manipulation of independent variables, control groups and randomization. On the other hand, if the researcher involves participation in the study as participant-observer with less control, qualitative research designs like exploratory design is recommended.

To evaluate a research design is whether the design enables the researcher to answer the research question conclusively. Substantively, the issue is whether the researcher selected a design that matches the aims of the research. For example, if the research purpose is descriptive or exploratory, an experimental design is not appropriate. Methodologically, the main design issue in quantitative studies is whether the research design provides the most accurate, unbiased, interpretable, and replicable evidence possible.

Author's Background

Pang Sze Sze, a year two student who is studying Master of Nursing in the Hong Kong Polytechnic University and the Hong Kong Sanatorium Hospital. (Email: szeszepang @yahoo.com)

Reference

Berglund, C.A. (2001). *Health Research*. Melbourne, Victoria: Oxford University Press.

Bowling, A. (2009). *Research Methods in Health: Investigating health and health services* (3rd ed.). Maidenhead, England: Open University Press.

Burns, N. & Grove, S.K. (2007). *Understanding Nursing Research: Building an evidence-based practice* (4th ed.). St. Louis: Saunders Elsevier.

Burns, N. & Grove, S.K. (2009). *The Practice of Nursing Research: Appraisal, Synthesis, and Generation of Evidence* (6th ed.). St. Louis: Saunders Elsevier.

Burnard, P. & Morrison, P. (1994). *Nursing Research in Action: Developing basic skills* (2nd ed.). Houndmills: Macmillan Press.

Cormack, D.F.S. & Benton, D.C. (1996). The research process. In: Cormack DFS (ed). *The Research Process in Nursing* (3rd ed.). Oxford: Blackwell Science.

Crookes, P. & Davies, S. (2004). *Research into Practice: Essential skills for reading and applying research in nursing and health* (2nd ed.). Philadelphia: Elsevier Ltd.

Denzin, N.K. (1989). *The research act: A theoretical introduction to sociological methods* (3rd ed.). New York: McGraw-Hill.

Dempsey, P.A. & Dempsey, A.D. (2000). *Using Nursing Research: Process, Critical Evaluation, and Utilization* (5th ed.). Philadelphia: Lippincott.

Draper, J. (2004). The relationship between research question and research design. *Research into Practice: Essential Skills for reading and applying research in nursing and health care*. Philadelphia: Elsevier Ltd.

Freshwater, D. & Bishop, V. (2004). *Nursing research in context: appreciation, application and professional development*. Houndmills: Palgrave Macmillan.

Gillis, A. & Jackson, W. (2002). *Research for Nurses: Methods and Interpretation*. Philadelphia: F.A. Davis Company.

Griffiths, F. (2009). *Research methods for health care practice*. London: Sage Publications Ltd.

Hek, G. & Moule, P. (2006). *Making sense of research: an introduction for health and social care practitioners*. London: Sage Publications Ltd.

Hicks, C. (2004). *Research methods for clinical therapists: applied project design and analysis* (4th ed.). London: Churchill Livingstone.

Holland, K. (1999). A journey to becoming: the student nurse transition. *Journal of Advanced Nursing,* 29(1), 229-336.

Hoskins, C.N. & Mariano, C. (2004). *Research in Nursing and Health: Understanding and Using Quantitative and Qualitative Methods* (2nd ed.). New York: Springer Publishing Company, Inc.

King, S.J. & Turner, S. (2000). Caring for adolescent females with anorexia nervosa: registered nurses' perspective. *Journal of Advanced Nursing*, 31(1), 139-147.

Levy, V. (1999). Protective steering: a grounded theory study of the processes by which midwives facilitate informed choices during pregnancy. *Journal of Advanced Nursing*, 29(1), 104-112.

Lobiondo-Wood, G. & Haber, J. (2009). *Nursing Research in Canada: Methods and Critical Appraisal for Evidence-Based Practice*. Canada: Mosby Elsevier.

Maltby, J., Williams, G., McGarry, J. & Day, L. (2010). *Research Methods for Nursing and Healthcare*. Harlow: Pearson Education Ltd.

Neale, J. (2009). *Research Methods for Health and Social Care*. Basingstoke: Palgrave Macmillan.

Neil, W. (2001). *The Health Project Book: A Handbook for new researchers in the field of health*. London: New York: Taylor & Francis.

Parahoo, K. (1997). *Nursing Research; Principles, Process and Issues*. Basingstoke: Macmillan.

Polit, D.F. & Hungler, B.P. (1991). *Nursing Research Principles and Methods* (4th ed.). Philadelphia: Lippincott.

Polit, D. & Beck, C. (2006). *Essentials of nursing research: methods, appraisal and utilization* (6th ed.). Philadelphia: Lippincott Williams and Wilkins.

Shi, L. (2008). *Health Services Research Methods* (2nd ed.). New York: Thomson Delmar Learning.

Stauss, A. & Corbin, J. (1990). *Basics of qualitative research: grounded theory procedures and techniques*. Newbury Park, CA: Sage Publications Inc.

Stem, E. (2005). *Evaluation research methods*. London: Sage Publication Ltd.

Smith, F., Francis, S.A. & Schafheutle, E. (2008). *International Research in Healthcare*. London: Pharmaceutical Press.

Weiss, M., Fawcett, J. & Aber, C. (2009). Adaptation, post-partum concerns, and learning needs in the first two weeks after caesarean birth. *Journal of Clinical Nursing*, 18(21), 2938-2948.

Wood, M.J. & Ross-Kerr, J.C. (2011) *Basic steps in planning nursing research: from question to proposal* (7th ed.). Sudbury: Jones and Bartlett.

In: Nursing Research: A Chinese Perspective
Editor: Zenobia C. Y. Chan

ISBN: 978-1-61209-833-3
©2011 Nova Science Publishers, Inc.

Chapter VII

Research Methods (Either Quantitative Research or Qualitative Research)

Janny Y. N. Chan and Zenobia C. Y. Chan
The Hong Kong Polytechnic University, China

Summary

Quantitative research is a numerical form of objective presentation. This paper focuses on the different types of research designs in which a nursing researcher would manipulate the entire picture into the quantitative research study. Each research designs has ve its own characteristics as well as pros and cons. It depends on how the research is structured and organized in a systematic ways for setting, sample or other variables that involved in the study.

Introduction

The portrait of research design involves abstractions such as the terms "happy" and "painful". These words are abstractions of human descriptive and subjective expressions that cannot be measured. The researcher is like a painter who may not able to express from what they have seen by doing nothing to let other know what is inside their mind. However, the painter could try to use their technique to interpretate an image or information. Sso, the painter or the researcher would make use of their colors and skills to illustrate in the picture. When we try to measure something that is measurable, we take quantitative research for achieving our objectives and interventions that would benefit future patient care and service. To gain the audiences' appreciation and recognition of the picture or the quantitative studies, we need to have the concepts that are called variables, such as weights and body temperature. Apart from of our purposeful interventions, we need to convince people among the comparable data so as to make the result more interpretable and concrete. Also, we need to equip our instruments and tools on how the data will be collected. A procedure is an art of collecting of data as there are many complexities of relationships among variables in which we need to control over it. It is just like the painter would make use of color contrast to make a clear standout of their objects. The number of times for the data collection should be well arranged for those there might be have changes over time. Setting is also an important for the outcome; such as whether you collect data from the community or the hospital, the range of data within the set may vary ies a lot. To conduct quantitative research, we need to consider some fundamental approaches, including its pros and cons in which we will cover in the following sections.

The Big Picture of Quantitative Research

According to Bulla (2010,p.26), it is necessary to clearly state the hypothesis, or the research question, before data collection starts. The well-established hypothesis is the backbone of reaching the goal of the research that could sum up to illustrate a phenomenon. The hypothesis or the research question plays an important role to identify whether it could voice out in front of other interest groups in a way that is relevant, credible, accurate, unbiased, and sensitive to the real situation in the community. Polit and Back (2010) states that it is a key to address in the design of quantitative study. Therefore, we need to decide if the hypotheses of the study could move stepping forward for an intervention. To strengthen the hypothesis, the researcher needs to make comparisons for interpreting results. It is like a portrait in which the painter is focusing at one object where the audience could view whether it is large or small comparing to the frame. Also, it is important to set some variables and controls for the entire research in order to prove the hypothesis. Besides, the sample sizes that involve in the research bind the set of data for a supportive and scientific reasoning for testing the hypothesis. Quantitative content analysis tends to be highly structured (Waltz, Strickland, & Lenz 2010). They states that there are three key inter-related processes involved: Conceptualizing and identifying characteristics of the content that are to be measured; determining the measures and explicit rules for identifying, coding, and recording the characteristics and sampling, coding, and tabulating the units (Waltz et al., 2010). In order to achieve the goal, time and places that the data will be collected is important to the design method. There is a timeframe when collecting the data in terms of its up-to-date fashion. Moreover, there are different types of designs of quantitative research – Experimental, quasi-experimental, and non-experimental designs.

1. Experimental Research

Experimental research is an active agent rather than a passive observer. The researcher takes part in the experiment for the valuable data from what they have seen, heard, smelled and touched. It is a common approach for the scientist who works in the laboratory where they could control it more easily. The Oobserver or the researcher could conduct research in any setting other than laboratory. The main qualification for an experimental design is to have three elements. There are manipulation, control and randomization. Manipulation is when the observer takes some actions with to the participants. The Ccontrol group is in used over the experimental setting because where variations occur to see the difference within. The experimenter could assign random participants to the group. The participants have the equal chance of being selected in any group. Sometimes, researchers would consider manipulating two or more variables simultaneously. It is called factorial design. It permits the testing of three hypotheses. In factorial experiments, subjects are assigned at random to a combination of treatments (Polit & Beck, 2010). Sometimes, the comparisons are between different people. When the same subjects are compared, the designs are within subjects' designs.

Pros and Cons of Experiment Research

Experiments are the most powerful designs for testing hypotheses of all cause and effect relationships because there is least amount of noise within the experiment and the control group is more consistent to manipulate. The outcome is somehow come very close to attaining the reality and facts. However, there are limitations for doing experiment design because the number of samples is random; therefore, it could not well present the whole conclusion well for specific human behaviors or characteristics. Ethical constraints are influence ing the outcome because the objective of the researcher may not be feasible to the subjects. Also, the Hawthorne effect may cause participants to change the behavior that is not realistic to the outcome or results. Therefore, it is difficult to apply experiments for real-world problems.

Table 1. The pros and cons of experimental, non-experimental, quasi-experimental, cross-sectional and longitudinal research designs

Research designs	Pros	Cons
Experimental	-Mmost powerful for testing hypotheses -Lleast noise -more consistent -more realistic	-random sample cannot present entire population -ethical constrains -participants change behavior due to Hawthorne effect
Non-experimental	-efficient of collecting large amount of data for correlation	-failure to state causal relationships with assurance -preexisted participants may have bias
Quasi-experimental	-more practical -easy to conduct in timeframe	-unwilling participation of subjects
Cross-sectional	-cheap -easy to manage	-inconsistent over time
Longitudinal	-more consistent data	-costly -difficult to control

2. Non-Experimental Research

There are some reasons to do the non-experimental research because the independent variable inherently cannot be manipulated or in which it would be unethical to manipulate the independent variable. There are two main types of the non-experimental research. One is called correlational designs and the other one is the retrospective design. A correlation is an inter-relationship between two variables and it could be detected through statistical analyses. For retrospective design, it is the comparative of the phenomena observed occurring in the past and in the present. Correlational studies with a prospective design start with a presumed cause and then go forward to the presumed effect. A second broad class of non-experimental studies is descriptive research. The purpose of descriptive studies is to observe, describe, and document aspects of a situation.

Pros and Cons of Non-Experimental Research

The major disadvantage of non-experimental research is that it cannot state the causal relationships with assurance. The Rresearcher works with pre-existing groups that may have bias for interpretive problems. However, correlational studies play a crucial role in nursing because many interesting problems are not amenable to experimentation. Correlation research is often an efficient and effective means of collecting a large amount of data about a problem (Polit & Beck, 2010).

3. Quasi-Experimental Research

According to Polit and Beck (2010, p.232), although intervention is involved, quasi-experimental designs weighs ts less on the randomization and control group may absence. As a nurse researcher, there are 2 commonly designs that are frequently used. One is the non-equivalent control group before-after design in which involves two or more groups of subjects observed before and after the implementation of an intervention. The other group is the Time-Series design. This would be used when there is an inability to obtain a meaningful control group. It involves data collection over a longer period of time, and ongoing there are is ongoing interventions within the period while data is still collected.

Pros and Cons of Quasi-Experimental Research

Quasi-experiment is more practical as a nurse could start an intervention within the data-collection timeframe. In fact, participants sometimes are not willing to be randomized in clinical trials. It is more likely to have the wider and broader group of people taking part in the quasi-experiment design, so as to make the result more generalized. The repeated measures over time for the same group of participants will be influenced by the sequence effects that will do affect the uncertainties in the outcome (Munro, Visintainer, & Page, 1986).

4. Cross-Sectional Research and Longitudinal Research

Researcher design in making their hypothesis is to decide when and how often the data will be collected. As stated by Polit and Back (2010, p.239), cross-sectional designs are the collection of data at one single point in time. All related phenomena in regards of the study are captured during one data collection period. Going back to our portrait of the picture, the painter only drew all of the fruits on the table in which have illustrated an image at the moment that he or she has viewed at the table. The fruits may deteriorate over couple of days so it is similar to describe the status of the phenomena or relationships among phenomena at a fixed point, for instance, the table and the fruits. Cross-sectional design is about associated with time. For the longitudinal designs, it plays a more persuasive role one from the cross-sectional design. The reason is because the object or the data source may have changed over time in responding to the questions. The respondents will have the different answers come up from the previous one that was been asked a few years ago. Perhaps it is the change of the conscious and educational level of the participant.

Pros and Cons of the Cross-Sectional and Longitudinal Research

As stated by Polit and Beck (2010, p.239), the pros of the cross-sectional design require sume lower cost and it is easier to manage. The cons are the change of time because it may influence the accuracy of data that could be valid for some years after. Therefore, longitudinal designs is with more consistent and applicable to the phenomena over years. For example, it will be more costly and difficult to control due to the mobility of that particular participant who was have interviewed years before.

Discussion and Application

Researchers choose a specific research study aimed s at the purpose and rationale in order to bring up interpretation. For example, by using some researcher's work - the study of feasibility and safety of a novel catheter-based and a permanent implant is good for avoiding stroke disease and for patients who are is not suitable for taking anticoagulants in terms of safety aspects (Katharinen et al., 2008). The researcher teams took experimental design for their study is because the results of the findings are obtained from the clinic and laboratories that could take close follow-up to patients who suffered in strokes with different treatments. The researchers take part in the experiment for the valuable data to test the hypothesis that is related to medication and the medical device.

For the non-experimental research, there is a paper that demonstrates the applications of methods of clinical epidemiology to problems in anesthesia and intensive care. The aims are to explore the quality of evidence to guide clinical decision-making and health policy by experimental and non-experimental designs as supplementary (Rigg, J.R.A., Jamrozik, K., & Myles, P.S., 1999). Ssince there are too many studies focusing on the risk factors and complications for post-operative surgery, and analyzing the problems for the morbidity of the perioperative factors. The independent variable, such as the patient who took a beta- blocker in reducing perioperative cardiac morbidity and mortality, inherently cannot be manipulated or there might be have some unethical issues in to manipulating e the independent variable. Thus, the authors took the non-experimental approach for obtaining a more intensive uncontrolled prospective survey. The data was to elaborate the understanding of a condition that provides high clinical and human cost to patients at postoperative surgery. This can provide important contributions to the understanding of prevention and management of complex problems such as advancement.

For the quasi-experimental research, there is a paper emphasizing that smoking is the risk factor of causing diseases. Many studies support to stopping smoking. S so, the authors established the objective to evaluate the effects of auricular acupressure combined with multimedia instruction in comparison with auricular acupressure alone on smoking cessation in young adults (Wang, Y.Z., Chen, H.H., & Yeh, M.L., 2010). The quasi-experimental research design was used in this episode. Some participants were assigned into two groups according to their preference of choosing which method for auricular acupressure. The results conclude that the combined intervention that involves both psychological and physical support was more effective than the auricular acupressure alone. The quasi-experimental research then could test the hypothesis by designing two interventions by two or three groups of subjects, such as the young smokers in this case, after a period of time to see whether which intervention is most efficient.

For aAn interesting paper that dedicates to cross-sectional research is about the measurement of newborn foot length to identify small babies in need of extra care (Marchant, T., Jaribu, J., Penfold, S., Tanner, M., & Armstrong, S.J., 2010). Since the researchers found that the neonatal mortality is due to low birth weight or prematurity remains high in many developing countries, they aimed to assess the sensitivity and specificity, and the predictive values of newborn foot length for identifying the low weight or premature babies. The researchers compare the foot sizes between the first day and the fifth day to determine if the baby is within the normal range of standard weight from an African hospital. They concluded that the measurement of newborn foot lengths could be an indicator for receiving palliative interventions and care for an improved survival. Therefore, it could be a guideline for most hospitals to follow-up when newborn's foot size is comparatively small in order to provide more intensive care to that baby selectively, especially for the overload of hospital occupancies that may decline the quality of health services that may cause a higher chance of unhealthy newborns after discharge from hospital.

For the longitudinal research, there is a paper about the acupuncture therapy in which the researchers investigate the experience and the effects of the course of acupuncture therapy. Samples of participants are all suffered from chronic illnesses that received s acupuncture therapy for the first time. The feedbacks was are well- defined as holistic as the treatment could improve the symptoms, energy, and personal and social identity. In this case, after the significant observations and data collection, it revealed s that acupuncture could be an alternative treatment for the chronic illness patient. This could promote the use of acupuncture in most developed countries where it is under some health insurance plans, such as in Canada, to improve patient's well being (Paterson & Britten, 2004).

Conclusion

Research is like a portrait. The painter or researcher could decide which instrument tools to express their views into the products for drawing the attentions of interest groups who ose have s not been explored and seen. It is the fantasy and juicy part of the creation that research consists. For different research approaches, like what I have given from the above researcher's works and papers, the preference of choosing the appropriate research design depending on the resources, settings and time in terms of the research questions that could influence the future quality of health service, quality of life and maximize the benefits for all mankind.

Author's Background

In preserving the high standards of research studies, the creative consideration for what we observe among changing phenomena would be an asset to future advancement in the healthcare service. Nurses should get involved ment and conduct their research and propose ing any implementation in clinical settings in order to improve human's well-being. Moreover, the research designs that I have been conducted are the basic idea of what research designs are available and for which circumstances to use them.

Chan Yan Nei, Janny Chan, a year two student who is studying Master of Nursing in the Hong Kong Polytechnic University. (Email: 09680392g@polyu.edu.hk)

References

Al-Atiyyat, N.M.H.(2008). Patient-related barriers to effective cancer pain management. *Journal of Hospice and Palliative Nursing*. 10(4), 198-204.

Burns, M., & Grove, S.K. (2005). *The practice of nursing research: Conduct, critique, and utilization* (5th ed.). St. Louis: Elsevier Saunders.

Chesnay, M.D., & Anderson, B.A. (2008). *Caring for the vulnerable: Perspectives in nursing theory, practice, and research* (2nd ed.). Sudbury: Jones and Bartlett Publishers.

Duffy, M. (2006). *A commonly encountered problem in quantitative research*. Lippincott Williams & Wilkins. 20(6), 273-276

Duffy, M.E. (2005). *Resources for critically appraising quantitative research evidence for nursing practice*. Lippinocott William & Wilkins, 19(5), 233-235.

Hulley, S.B., Cummings, S.R., Browner, W.S., Grady, D.G., & Newman, T.B. (2007). *Designing clinical research* (3th ed.). Philadelphia: Lippincott Williams & Wilkins.

Katharinen, S., & Israel, C. (2008). A novel endovascular device for emboli re-routing: Part I: Evaluation in a swine model. *Stroke*, 39(10):2860-2866.

Legare, F., Stewart, M., Frosch, D., Grimshaw, J., Labrecque, M., & Magnan, M. (2009). Exackte(2): Exploiting the clinical consultation as a knowledge transfer and exchange environment: a study protocol. *Implementation Science*. 4,14

Marchant, T., Jaribu, J., Penfold, S., Tanner, M., & Armstrong, S.J. (2010). Measuring newborn foot length to identify small babies in need of extra care: a cross- sectional hospital- based study with community follow-up in Tanzania. *BMC Public Health.* 10:624, 2010.

Martin, C.R., & Thompson, D.R. (2000). *Design and analysis of clinical nursing research studies* (1st ed.). London: Routledge.

Mattila, E., Kaunonen, M., Aalto, Pirjo., Ollikainen, Jyrki., & Astedt-Kurki, P. (2010). Support for hospital patients and associated factors. *Scandinavian Journal of Caring Sciences.* 24, 734-745

McLaughlin, M.M., & Bulla, S.A. (2010). *Real nursing research: The quest for magnet recognition.* Sudbury: Jones and Bartlett Publishers.

Munro, B.H., Visintainer, M.A., & Page, E.B. (1986). *Statistical methods for health care research.* Philadelphia: J.B. Lippincott Company.

Paterson, C., & Britten, N. (2004). Acupuncture as a complex intervention: A holistic model. *Journal of Alternative & Complementary Medicine.* 10(5), 791-801.

Polit, D.F., & Beck, C.T. (2010). *Essentials of nursing research: Appraising evidence for nursing practice* (7th ed.). Philadelphia: Lippinocott Williams & Wilkins.

Rigg, J.R.A., Jamrozik, K., & Myles, P.S. (1999). Evidence-based methods to improve anaesthesia and intensive care. *Current Opinion in Anaesthesiology,* Vol.12(2), 221-227.

Verduin, F., Scholte, W.F., Rutayisire, T., & Richters, A. (2010). How qualitative information helped to shape quantitative research instruments in rRwanda. *Intervention,* 8(3), 233-244.

Waltz, C.F., Strickland, O.L., & Lenz, E.R. (2010). *Measurement in nursing and health research* (4th ed.). New York: Springer Publishing Company, LLC

Wang, Y.Z., Chen, H.H., & Yeh, M.L. (2010). Auricular acupressure combined with multimedia instruction or alone for quitting smoking in young adults: A quasi-experimental study. *International Journal of Nursing Studies,* 47(9), 1089-95.

Wing, S., Horton, R.A., Muhammad, N., Grant, G.R., Tajik, M., & Thu, Kendall. (2008). Integrating epidemiology, education, and organizing for environmental justice: Community health effects of industrial hog operations. *American Journal of Public Health,* 98 (8), 1390-1397.

In: Nursing Research: A Chinese Perspective
Editor: Zenobia C. Y. Chan

ISBN: 978-1-61209-833-3
©2011 Nova Science Publishers, Inc.

Chapter VIII

Beginning of Survey: Principle Questions, Data Variables and Different Types

Steve S. C. Wong and Zenobia C. Y. Chan
The Hong Kong Polytechnic University, China

Summary

There are many types of data collection methods in quantitative research. Data collection is of utmost important in the research process since it can cause a chain of problems if a wrong data collection method is used. Inappropriate sampling and irrelevant data and information will be collected if a wrong data collection method is employed. Therefore, this paper aims to introduce you to the importance of data collection in the research process. After knowing the importance of data collection, this paper will further discuss a type of data collection method – survey – used in quantitative research method. The second part of this paper will introduce you to some optimal questions needed to know before using a survey, and the different variables used in a survey and different types of surveys. Advantages and disadvantages of each type of survey are also discussed in this paper. Finally, Tthe paper finally will briefly explain the recent trend of using Internet survey as a powerful data collection tool.

Introduction

It is not surprising that research is part of our daily life. There are thousands of researches conducted or in processing that can be used to describe a person's behavior or to provide opinions and indexes on daily issues and activities, such as an evaluation of a commodity or a report discussing the latest policy address from the Government. Research is to answer questions through scientific methods (Wrench, Thomas-Maddox, Richmond, & McCroskey, 2008). A more simple definition of research is from Keyton (2006) which introduces research ias the process of asking questions and looking for answers. Therefore, you and I actually are conducting numerous researches every day. For example, you may ask your friends' opinions or suggestions on a movie that you are interested in. Then, you consolidate all different opinions and suggestions from your friends. Finally, you decide to watch or not to watch the movie from the gathered opinions. This is only a single example of research, regardless of its informal manner, that people conduct in their daily life.

A formal, or in other words, an academic research involves a couples of steps. There are many types of research approaches. The most common approach that people come across in their daily real life situation is communication research, which is conducted by communication scholars to discover communication phenomena by employing qualitative or quantitative research methods, of which both of them are empirical, which means they are based on observations or experiences; the difference between these two methods is that qualitative is more subjective while quantitative is more objective (Keyton, 2006). The following two short paragraphs will briefly explain their characteristics.

Qualitative research method focuses on locating the complexity of communication phenomena. As Lindlof & Taylor discussed, qualitative research maintains the form and content of human activities or interactions in a way of text which is then analyzed for the quality (as cited in Keyton, 2006, p. 59). Since qualitative grounds on the content of human activities and interactions, this research method highly depends on the experiences of interviewees or participants. And, inductive analysis, moving from specific to general, is another feature of qualitative research method (Keyton, 2006). Therefore, qualitative method gives researchers a subjective data. After collecting data from different interviewees or participants, researchers will then analyze and discuss the collected data and information. In general, qualitative research method includes interviews, focus groups, narrative analyseis and participant observations (Priest, 2010).

In contrast, quantitative research method relies on numbers rather than on text. Quantitative research is concerned s with about numbers and statistics (Bradley, 2010). Precisely, quantitative researchers apply measurement and observation to represent communication phenomenon as amounts, frequencies, degrees, values, or intensity (Keyton, 2006). Quantitative analysis employs a deductive approach. Deductive analysis is totally opposite from inductive analysis in that deductive analysis discusses things from general (theory) to specific (research conclusion), that is, quantitative researchers aim at verifying if what the theory proposed is to be correct (Keyton, 2006). Objectivity is preserved in quantitative method since it highly depends on numerical data. Surveys and experiments are some examples of quantitative research methods (Priest, 2010).

It is expected that you have a general picture among qualitative and quantitative researches after a brief introduction of both methods. However, this paper will mainly focus on discussing surveys, which are is a types of data collection methods of quantitative. As surveys are is widely used in clinical settings, this paper will heavily explain some special characteristics of a survey. The remaining part of this paper will give you a discussion of the general importance of data collection, followed by discussing some basic questions researchers have to understand before conducting a survey, different types of variable applied in a survey, and the trend of using a web-based survey and the related benefits and costs.

The Importance of Data Collection

Every research requires a series of processes to be accomplished. For example, you have to consider the planning, preparation and statistical concept, as well as discussing and interpreting the of statistical analysis in a quantitative research (Thompson, Schwartz, Davis, & Panacek, 1996). There are a couples of components inside this series, for example, forming a research question, deciding on the choice of data collection method, and evaluating the research result. However, the process of data collection is termed to be the utmost important part amongst this series. According to Maltby, Williams, McGarry, & Day (2010), data collection is a research component that has to be decided before the research starts since it affects the sampling process and the ability to answer the research questions that is preset. In another words, research questions cannot be answered if aa wrong or improper data collection method is employed since the data or variables that collected may not be appropriated in answering towards the research questions. Moreover, data collection methods and sampling are interrelated. For example, a focus group requires the candidates to share some similar interests, such as they suffer from same disease, while a simple phone-interview may not need any prerequisites on candidates. If the phone-interview is wrongly selected for a research on treatment prognosis of a designated disease, it is definitely that the research will fail in answering the research questions, and the research is termed as not reliable and not valid.

Optimal Questions to be asked Before Conducting a Survey

As mentioned before, only survey will be introduced in this paper. A Ssurvey is a collection tool that is used to gather data and information of people about their personal particulars, such as education and finance status, and their beliefs and behaviors on some issues (Balnaves & Caputi, 2001). A Ssurvey can be done in a format of a questionnaire, and it is composed of by different types of variables.

Now you have already got the general idea of the importance of data collection and what a survey is,. Iit is the time for researchers to ask themselves whether a survey is the best data collection method to be applied in their research. Assuming you are going to use a survey as your collection tool, however, you have to ask three basic questions before you really start the data collection process (Wrench et al., 2008). The first question that a researcher has to ask is what data and information he/she wants to get. This is important for researchers as he/she can eliminate any inappropriate data, and spend more time to focusing on the ose valuable data that can best answer the preset research questions. The second question for researchers is that whether there is a need to collect new data, that is, are there any researches done before that are similar to yours one. It is You are expected that you will get similar data and information as previous researches if your topic is more or less the same as before. The last question for researchers to consider is whether the interviewees understand anything about your research. For example, you are interested in the drug tamiflu that is used to treat H_1N_1;, the first question you have to ask yourself is what aspects of question you want to discover, such as the effectiveness, the side effects or the cost of tamiflu. If you are going to explore the level of effectiveness of tamiflu, you have to explore as well if there are is any previous researches that already discussed on such an issue. If no previous researches have been made, then you step forward to consider your interviewees if they know or are familiar with what tamiflu is. It is obvious that irrelevant data and information will be collected if you go to interview people who did not suffer from H_1N_1 or people who have suffered from but have recovered without any medication.

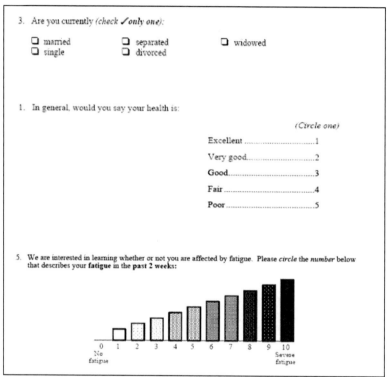

Source: Stanford Patient Education Research Center, Stanford University School of Medicine, n.d.

Figure 1. Extract of questions from diabetes survey.

Different Variables used in Survey

There are mainly three types of variables used in a survey;, namely, nominal, ordinal and interval. A Nnominal variable is designed to describe data in categorical form (Balnaves & Caputi, 2001). In other words, data of a nominal variable can be viewed as distinct from one and other (Maltby et al., 2010). That is, the data itself is themselves are physically not the same, however, they can be put into the same category. Gender is the most suitable example of a nominal variable. Another example of a nominal variable is marital status as shown in Fig. 1 question 3. Those five marital statuses are individually independent, however, all of them can be grouped under the same category – marital status. Ordinal variable, on the other hand, is a type of variable that requires interviewees to respondse in rank order (Balnaves &

Caputi, 2001). Pain score used in clinical settings to evaluate the level of pain of patients is a kind of ordinal variable. Patients are asked to give a score, from 0 (no pain) to 10 (very painful), to indicate their level of pain.

The numbers used here do not have any numerical value, that is, the 0-10 score is just only a reflection of the level of pain, whereas there is no equal difference between 0 (painless), 1 (less pain), and 2 (little pain) and so forth (Maltby et al., 2010). Question 5 in Fig. 1 is another example of an ordinal variable. The fatigue level is more or less the same as the pain score that patients are asked to make a decision on either the level of pain or fatigue, of which the numbers themselves are meaningless and there is none equal discrepancy between any two numbers. A Ffeature of an interval variable is similar to that of an ordinal variable. Numbers or wordings in interval variables have a meaning of retrogression and progression. Take the same example in Fig. 1, the question that is asking for health status offers five progressive interval variables. Nevertheless, they look like ordinal variables, each of them possesses an equal difference. The difference between "Very good" (2), "Good" (3) and "Fair" (4) is obvious and the interval between them is said to be equal.

Types of Survey and their Trend

There are numerous types of surveys, such as an interview survey, a telephone survey, a mail survey and a web-based survey, available in the research field. Each of them has their own advantages and disadvantages, which will be discussed in the following.

An Iinterview survey requires the existence of one or more professional interviewers to conduct the interview. As face-to-face between interviewers and interviewees is required in an interview survey, therefore, a proper environment is needed in order to perform the interview. The environment should be comfortable and with suitable lighting, as well as quiet enough so that the interview will not be disturbed from outside noise. It is said that interview surveys would generate a higher response rate than other types of surveys as the presence of interviewers can minimize the chance of "don't know" answers through the persistence and professional questioning skill of the by interviewer (Tourangeau, 2003; Babbie, 2011), and the interview survey offers one advantage that other methods could not offer, that is body language. Body language offers additional information of interviewees' mood and attitude that verbal communication cannot provide. Moreover, interviewers can offer assistance to interviewees who have difficulty in answering the questions. However, an interview survey does have drawbacks to the research team. The cost is very high for an interview survey as it needs well-trained interviewers and the arrangement of a proper place to conduct the interview. Time is also one of the concerns since the interview time is mutually compromised between interviewers and interviewees.

Another type of survey is the telephone survey, which is conducted through the telephone instead of a face-to-face interview. The benefit of using telephone is that it is more cost effective as there is no need for the arrangement of an interview place and the presence of professional interviewers. In addition to, telephone survey can reach more targeted interviewees as it is supposed that everyone has gets a cell phone nowadays (Babbie, 2011). Telephone surveys can even reach overseas interviewees, that is, the telephone survey is not restricted by geographical distance. However, the timing of a telephone survey is difficult to control since the interviewees may not be free when answering the phone. And, interviewees may just provide superficial answers as they want to hang up as soon as possible.

Mail surveys, nowadays, are used has less frequently use by researchers because of its numerous drawbacks. As mMail surveys takes a longer time and are more expensive than other types of surveys to reach to interviewees, and there is always a chance of mis-delivery of the survey. Moreover, the response rate is comparatively low since interviewees can just ignore and neglect the mail survey without sending it back or even throwing it away. Sending a self-addressed stamped envelope together with the mail survey is a normal practice to increase the response rate (Wrench et al., 2008).

Web-based surveys or Internet surveys are is the most recent type of surveys in this century. This is because Internet usage is more popular nowadays, and the Internet can reach almost every single city or place around the world. It is said that the use of an Internet survey can speed up the delivery and receiving time of the survey, and the wide coverage of the Internet ensures the survey can reach larger amounts of targeted interviewees (Wharton, Hampl, Hall, & Winham, 2003). The risk of mis-delivery or prolonged postal time is eliminated as every survey is sentding to and from Internet, unless there is a problem on the Internet server. Besides, the research cost can be kept as low as possible since there is no need for a interview place and trained interviewers. The cost is also saved through the unnecessary printing expenses as all the materials are developed and transmitted electronically. In addition, visual aids, such as diagrams and video clips can be added in the Internet survey without extra cost to make the survey being more informative, comprehensive and attractive (Tourangeau, 2003). Apart from these advantages, there are several disadvantages of Internet survey. Internet survey may not be a proper data collection method if the targeted interviewees are the elderly, who have s inadequate knowledge ofn computers and using the Internet. And, sSecurity is also a main concern for Internet survey. As the Internet can be accessed anywhere and anytime once you have the login code of Eemail, confidentiality may not be fully protected. However, this can be managed by adding a security code on the file (Wharton et al., 2003). Last but not the least, the difference of web browsers between researchers and interviewees may also cause a problem as the materials of the survey may not be seen at the interviewees' computers. This can be resolved by editing the Internet survey with lowest common denominator of computer sophistication (Wharton et al., 2003).

The use of Internet surveys have s been increasincreasing ed during these decades. This increasing trend of usage is primarily due to the increased popularity of the Internet and the ease of access of the Internet. Different tools of advanced technology have been applied to Internet surveys such as Eemail, the conventional tool, and personal digital assistant (PDA). It is confirmed that the timing to complete, data input of a PDA-based survey is much lesser and the cost of performing the PDA-based survey is also reduced (Yu, Courten, Pan, Galea, & Pryor, 2009). However, the Internet survey is a kind of self-administered survey, that is the interviewees receive and complete the survey without assistance from interviewers (Wrench et al., 2008). The lack of support from researchers is a problem if interviewees do not understand the questions being asked (Wrench et al., 2008). It is suggested that researchers should add their contact information inside the Internet survey in order to provide a channel in case interviewees have any difficulties in answering the survey. Nevertheless, the Internet survey is still a valuable data collection method as it saves research budget and covers a larger population of interviewees to enhance the trustworthiness of the researches. And, using the

Internet survey is more environmental friendly to the community as none papers are used during the delivery and receiving period.

Author's Background

Wong Siu Chung, Steve,Steve Wong is studying in Master of Nursing in Hong Kong Polytechnic University after his first business degree. He wishes to pursue a career in nursing to help the ill people during the suffering period. (Email: steve_wong618@hotmail.com)

Siu Chung Steve Wong, (Email: steve_wong618@hotmail.com)

References

Babbie, E. (2011). *Introduction to social research.* Belmont, Calif. : Wadsworth/Cengage Learning.

Balnaves, M., & Caputi, P. (2001). *Introduction to quantitative research methods : an investigative approach.* London : SAGE.

Beebe, T. J., Locke III, G. R., Barnes, S. A., Davern, M. E., & Anderson, K. J. (2007). Mixing web and mail methods in a survey of physicians. *Health Services Research, 42*(3), 1219-1234.

Bradley, N. (2010). *Marketing research : tools & techniques.* Oxford ; New York : Oxford University Press.

Cantrell, M. A., & Lupinacci, P. (2007). Methodological issues in online data collection. *Journal of Advanced Nursing, 60*(5), 544-549.

Keyton, J. (2006). *Communication research : asking questions, finding answers.* New York : McGraw-Hill.

Maltby, J., Williams, G., McGarry, J., & Day, L. (2010). *Research methods for nursing and healthcare.* Harlow : Pearson Education.

Phillips, P. P., & Stawarski, C. A. (2008). *Data collection : planning for and collecting all types of data.* San Francisco, Calif. : Pfeiffer.

Priest, S. H. (2010). *Doing media research : an introduction.* Los Angeles : Sage.

Sapsford, R., & Jupp, V. (1996). *Data collection and analysis.* London ; Thousand Oaks, Calif. : Sage in association with Open University.

Schneider, J. K., & Deenan, A. (2004). Reducing quantitative data errors: tips for clinical researchers. *Applied Nursing Research, 17*(2), 125-129.

Stanford Patient Education Research Center, Stanford University School of Medicine. (n.d.). *Sample questionnaire – diabetes.* Retrieved on November 20, 2010 from http://patienteducation.stanford.edu/research/diabquest.pdf.

Tarbox, J., Wilke, A. E., Findel-Pyles, R. S., Bergstrom, R. M., Granpeesheh, D. (2010). A comparison of electronic to traditional pen-and-paper data collection in discrete trial training for children with autism. *Research in Autism Spectrum Disorders, Vol. 4,* 65-75.

Taylor, G. R. (2005). *Integrating quantitative and qualitative methods in research.* Lanham, Md. : University Press of America.

Thompson, C. B., Schwartz, R., Davis, E., & Panacek, E. A. (1996). Basics of research (part 6): quantitative data analysis. *Air Medical Journal, 15*(2), 73-84.

Tourangeau, R. (2003). Survey research and societal change. *Annual Review of Psychology, 55,* 775-801.

VanderStoep, S. W., & Johnston, D. D. (2009). *Research methods for everyday life : blending qualitative and quantitative approaches.* San Francisco, CA : Jossey-Bass.

Wharton, C. M., Hampl, J. S., Hall, R., & Winham, D. M. (2003). Pcs or paper-and-pencil: online surveys for data collection. *Journal of the American Dietetic Association, 103*(11), 1458-1459.

Wrench, J. S., Thomas-Maddox, C., Richmond, V. P., & McCroskey, J. C. (2008). *Quantitative research methods for communication : a hands-on approach.* New York, N.Y.: Oxford University Press.

Yu, P., Courten, M. D., Pan, E., Galea, G., & Pryor, J. (2009). The development and evaluation of a pda-based method for public health surveillance data collection in developing countries. *International Journal of Medical Informatics, 78,* 532-542.

In: Nursing Research: A Chinese Perspective
Editor: Zenobia C. Y. Chan

ISBN: 978-1-61209-833-3
©2011 Nova Science Publishers, Inc.

Chapter IX

Believe It or Not: Sampling Makes Quantitative Research Easy

Zoey S. S. Lam and Zenobia C. Y. Chan
The Hong Kong Polytechnic University, China

Summary

Sampling is the process of selecting individuals that represent the population, so that the result obtained from a study can be generalized to that population. This paper focuses on and compares the probability and non-probability sampling strategies used in the quantitative research. Although simple random sampling is said to be the gold standard for quantitative studies, it is rarely adopted due to its cost and complexity. Other modified forms such as stratified sampling, cluster sampling, and systemic sampling are used instead. Though quantitative studies focus on the generalizability of the findings, which the probability sampling can fulfill, non-probability sampling is common in nursing researches. Therefore, it is very important to understand the rationales behind both probability and non-probability samplings in order to decide whether the findings of a study can be applied to a specific group of people. In addition to the kinds of sampling techniques, sample size, sampling error and sampling bias will be briefly discussed as well. This aims to provide a detailed picture of the sampling procedure in the quantitative research.

Introduction

When a research is being done, one starts with a problem that exists in a population. Population, or sometimes refers as target population, is the entire group of people that can possibly be included in the study (Macnee & McCabe, 2008). It doeis not only restricted to human subjects, but may include an entire set of objects, events, or elements that the researcher is interested in looking at (Bowling, 2002).or aA subset of the target population to which the researcher has reasonable access to is study population (Hulley, Cummings, Browner, Grady, & Newman, 2007). When a subgroup of individuals is selected from the study population, the term is called a sample (Tulchinsky & Varavikova, 2009). Unless the population size is extremely small, it is not possible for researchers to study every individual within the potential population (Macnee & McCabe, 2008). Therefore, sampling is an inevitable procedure in any researches. As a sample is selected for a study, researchers need to ensure that the sample is representative of the larger population, so that generalizations can be made about the entire population when characteristics of the sample are determined after conducting the research (Scott & Morrison, 2006). Since it is not feasible to expect the entire population to participate in a study, sampling is therefore an accepted alternative.

Sampling is the process of choosing individuals for a study, and that individuals being selected represent the larger group from which they come from (Fain, 2004). In other words, the purpose of sampling is to ensure that the characteristics of interest are likely to be present in all of the subjects being studied (Macnee & McCabe, 2008). With an involvement of a representative sample, researchers are in greater confidence to draw conclusions from the sample findings that are generalizable to the population (Stommel & Wills, 2004). Furthermore, studying a small number of subjects not only makes data collection more efficient, but also less costly and potentially more accurate (Polit & Beck, 2004). However, some concerns may arise due to the risk of potential bias in the process of selection (McGlynn, 1998). As a consequence of improper sampling, error in interpretation of results occurs, and this decreases the ability to generalize the findings beyond the subjects actually studied.

Before researchers prepare to recruit study subjects, it is crucial to define and describe the population, and specifically stipulate a sampling frame. A Ssampling frame is a list of the sampling elements in the target population (Scott & Morrison, 2006). It serves as a basis to decide whether an individual would be classified as a member of the population in question (Brink & Walt, 2006). To determine the way that the participants are to be selected, a set of inclusion and exclusion criteria has to be formulated to define a fairly homogeneous sample so that the extraneous variables are controlled (Houser, 2008). All persons with characteristics enlisted in the inclusion criteria will be recruited in the sample (Macnee & McCabe, 2008). Most of the time, population is also defined in terms of exclusion criteria, which is a list of characteristics that people must not possess (Polit & Beck, 2004). When subjects who meet the inclusion criteria but must be excluded, either because they cannot complete the study or they possess unique characteristics that may confound the results, exclusion criteria will be applied (Houser, 2008).

Although sampling, as describes so far, seems to be a complex process, it is actually a familiar procedure that we adopt everyday through our daily activities (Houser, 2008). We gather knowledge, make decisions, and formulate predictions based on sampling procedure (Wood & Haber, 2006). Not only that, scientists and other professions, derive knowledge through the same process. Also, nursing professions, who acquire skills of evidence-based practice in clinical settings, integrate their understanding of sampling into practices. To ensure that the clinical problem addressed by a study can be applicable to the right group of patients, it is necessary to understand the implications of different sampling techniques (Macnee and McCabe, 2008). Therefore, learning different types of sampling techniques is not only important to researchers, but also to the readers, who make judgments and integrate the research findings into practice. In this paper, emphasis will be stressed on the probability and non-probability sampling techniques employed in the quantitative research. Other factors related to sampling, such as sample size, sampling error and sampling bias will be discussed as well.

Types of Sampling

There are two broad categories of sampling methods. They are probability and non-probability samplings. The choice of sampling depends whether the selection involves randomization (Macnee and McCabe, 2008), or whether there is a sampling frame available (Fain, 2004). Table 1 summarizes the features of both the probability and non-probability samplings in quantitative research.

Table 1. Features of probability and non-probability samplings.

Probability Sampling	Non- Probability Sampling
- Individuals in population have equal chance to be selected	- Individuals in population are not selected randomly
- Process is complex, costly and not feasible	- Process is more practical to carry out
- Findings can be generalized to larger population	- Less likely to produce accurate and representative samples
- Sampling frame is required	- No sampling frame
- Sample size is determined by statistical analysis	- Sample size is not pre-determined, and is depended on the achievement of saturation

Types of Probability Sampling

The four most common types of probability sampling are simple random sampling, stratified sampling, cluster sampling, and systemic sampling. Simple random sampling is by far the purest form of probability sampling. Each member of the population has an equal chance of being selected (Wallen & Fraenkle, 2001). However, when the population is very large, it is often difficult and impossible to identify every member of the population. Therefore, systematic sampling may be used. Upon calculating, the required sample size for the study, every k^{th} individual, which k is the sampling interval, is selected from a list of population members (Gustavsson, 2007). Although systematic sampling is not claimed to be a strictly probability sampling, it is believed that this technique is as good as the random sampling method if the list of population members does not contain any hidden orders (Polit

& Beck, 2004). Owing to its simplicity, systematic sampling is put at a greater advantage over random sampling most of the time.

Stratified sampling, which is another commonly used probability method in research, minimizes the errors in sampling by subdividing the population into homogenous subsets, called strata (Wood and Haber, 2006). Each stratum consists of individuals that shares at least one common characteristic, such as gender, age, and occupation (Burns & Grove, 2005). By identifying the relevant strata and their actual representation in the population, random sampling can then be used to select a sufficient number of subjects from each stratum. However, one drawback from this method is that the stratifying attributes have to be known in advance and that the attributes may not be readily discernible (Polit & Beck, 2004). The forth and also the most complex sampling technique in quantitative research is cluster sampling. This technique involves multiple stages of sampling (Stommel & Wills 2004). By integrating either random or stratified methods in this sampling, the researcher is able to achieve a rich variety of results that are useful in different context (Macnee and McCabe, 2008). This type of method is used particularly when the population is very large and widely dispersed because of its convenience (Hulley et al., 2007). An example is the study conducted by Chen et.al (2005), which examines the public health nurses' knowledge of osteoporosis and its related factors in Taiwan during 2000. Because the study covered all the of he public health nurses in Taiwan's health centers, including those rural and mountain areas, cluster sampling was thereby employed by the researchers. In Table 2, the advantages and disadvantages of each type of probability sampling are listed.

Table 2. Advantages and disadvantages of probability sampling methods.

Probability Sampling	Advantages	Disadvantages
Random Sampling	- Eliminate likelihood of systematic bias in the sample - Results are more generalized	- Time consuming - Costly
Stratified Sampling	- Same as random sampling	- Same as random sampling
Cluster Sampling	- Same as random sampling, but more efficient - More economical and practical to carry out when population is widely dispersed	- The elements that subdivide the population into strata, must be know before random selection.
Systemic Sampling	- Easy to conduct - Able to yield the same result as random sampling method	- May have bias when the individuals with variables of interest are listed in the same interval as the sampling interval

Types of Non-Probability Sampling

Although the use of non-probability samples in most quantitative studies is problematic, they are used in most nursing studies due to its convenience and economic reasons (Macnee and McCabe, 2008). The three commonly used methods include convenience sampling, quota sampling and purposive sampling. Convenience sampling makes use of most conveniently available people as study subjects (Scott & Morrison, 2006). Though the subjects are readily approachable, some might be atypical of the population of interest, leading to bias in the sampling (Polit & Beck, 2004). However, it is still used in researches, which the sampling bias can be compromised. This is demonstrated by Callaghan (1999), who investigated the relationship between the nurses' health belief and their health- related behaviors in the United Kingdom. Regardless of the convenience sampling was used, the sampling bias was minimized as researchers found that the sample groups selected were similar to the study population at two different institutions in terms of the age, gender ratio and areas of nursing practice. Therefore, the sample chosen is said to be more representative to the population of interest in this case.

Table 3. Advantages and disadvantages of non-probability sampling methods.

Non- Probability Sampling	Advantages	Disadvantages
Convenience Sampling	- Inexpensive - Easier to recruit subjects	- No control over factors that will introduce bias to study - Generalizability is difficult
Quota Sampling	- Researcher can control the sample on selected characteristics - Sample is more closely resembles the population of interest	- Systematic variations - Bias in sample is possible
Purposive Sampling	- Able to locate sample that is hard to identify	- The greater the sample is limited by selected characteristics the less likely it is to generalize

Quota sampling is very similar to the stratified probability sampling (Burns & Grove, 2005). However, the only difference is that quota sampling is the selection of a non- random sample, which the researchers have control over who will be in the sample (Fain, 2004). Like convenience sampling, subjects in quota sampling are convenience samples from each population stratum (Burns & Grove, 2005). Although quota sampling is a relatively simple technique and it enhances the representativeness of a non-probability sample, many researchers fail to consider the benefits of this technique while planning a research (Polit & Beck, 2004). Lastly, when the target population is rare or difficult to locate, purposive sampling will be the only option (Swanson and Hilton, 2005). In this approach, individuals are selected based on the particular purpose of the experiment. An Eexample is the study which explores the choices and constraints experienced by registered mental nurses in obtaining the first post after qualification (Robinson and Murrells, 1998). Instead of taking all mental nurse students into study, the researcher purposively selected those that undergo the traditional program for qualification. Through this technique, the researcher not only focused on a particular characteristic, such as traditional program, but could also make a comparison on the choice and constraints experienced by people who graduated from the traditional program and those from newly launched educational programs. Table 3 shows the advantages and disadvantages of each type of non-probability sampling techniques.

Probability versus Non-Probability Samplings

While there are a variety of sampling methods available for quantitative research, it is not easy to say which of the particular method works best for a study as each of them has its own features. Probability sampling, as many textbooks imply, is an ideal procedure to ensure the representativeness of a study population (Wood and Haber, 2006). Since quantitative researchers aim to select a sample that enables them to generalize their findings to much broader groups, probability samplings clearly are the possible option. Though non-probability sampling is cheap and less complex, it is more likely to introduce bias into a sample, thereby making the representativeness of the population of interest less possible (Polit & Beck 2004). Due to the lack of generalizability, non-probability sampling is not often used in quantitative research (Fox, Hunn and Mathers, 2009). Since qualitative researchers are not concerned with the issues of generalizability but seek to select a sample that allows for an in-depth understanding of the phenomenon of interest, such techniques are more commonly found in qualitative research (Burns & Grove, 2005). This may be a reason why some of the textbooks either fail to introduce the methods of non-probability sampling under the chapter of quantitative research or refer them as a sampling technique used only in qualitative research.

Sample Size

While sample selection determines whether results can be generalized, the size of the sample affects whether the results can be trusted (Hoiser, 2008). In quantitative research, sample size is driven by the goal of generalizability (Wood and Haber, 2006). According to Macnee & McCabe (2008), probability samples often can be smaller than the non-probability samples because the former controls bias through random selection. Non-probability samples must be larger, on the other hand, as any biases caused by systemic factors can be cancelled out by the number of subjects. Though it tends to be a general rule that the bigger the sample the more accurate the findings in quantitative research, researchers have to ensure that the sample size is manageable owing to the time and resource constraints (Dawson, 2002). Power analysis is a strategy that enables quantitative researchers to determine the size of sample needed to detect a true relationship under study (Macnee and McCabe, 2008). While this test provides researchers with the minimum number of subjects to be included in the sample, various factors that affect sample size requirements in quantitative studies have to be considered. For instance, a small sample is considered adequate if the population is relatively homogenous, the dependent and independent variables are strongly related, or the measuring tools are precise and not prone to errors (Polit & Beck 2004). However, if attrition is a problem or a sample is divided to test for subgroup effects, a larger size than the estimated sample size will be needed for the study (Stommel & Wills, 2004). This is why, it is very important for the researchers to put the overall picture in mind and consider any potential factors that will influence the sample size.

Sampling Error and Sampling Bias

As McGlynn (1998) mentioned, even with a well-designed research, any results for a population based on a random sample may still contain sampling bias and error. Sampling errors occurs because only subgroups of individuals are randomly sampled. However, this type of error can be decreased by increasing the sample size. That means, the larger the sample and the more homogenous the population, the smaller is the sampling error results (Brink and Walt, 2006). In a mathematical sense, the minimization of sampling errors is proportional to the square root of the sample size (McGlynn, 1998). Sampling bias, on the other hand, is a systematic tendency to overestimate or underestimate the sample (Houser, 2008). This can be introduced by the researcher when the sample is not completely randomly selected (Brink & Walt, 2006). Nevertheless, this is a common problem associates with non-probability sampling, and the problem can be resolved by modifying the way in which the sample is being selected.

Conclusion

In quantitative research, sampling is an essential component that influences the meaning of the result. As mentioned above, several factors need to be considered before drawing the sample from a population. These include the nature or the goal of study, the accessibility of subjects and the size of sample. In order to generalize the findings from sample to population, probability sampling is needed to ensure the sample is representative to the population which they select from. However, when generalization is less important, non-probability sampling can be considered. Non-probability sampling allows researchers to yield very useful information if the subjects are selected thoughtfully. Unfortunately, this is not often the purpose of quantitative research. Nevertheless, non-probability samples are still used in many nursing researches because of their skills and resources involved. Therefore, when one is reading a research paper, he/ she should be cautious as to decide whether the finding is applicable to other populations, or groups of patients.

Author's Background

Lam Shan Shan, Zoey, who graduated from the Bachelor of Science program in pharmacology, is now studying Master of Nursing in the Hong Kong Polytechnic University and the Hong Kong Sanatorium Hospital. (Email: shanshan_lam@hotmail.com)

References

Bowling, A. (2002). *Research methods in health: Investigating health and health services.* (2nd ed.). Open University Press: Buckingham.

Brink, H., & Walt, C. V. D. (2006). *Fundamentals of Research Methodology for Healthcare Professionals.* (2nd ed.). Berne Convention: Lansdowne.

Callaghan, P. (1999). Health beliefs and their influence on United Kingdom nurses' health-related behaviours. *Journal of Advanced Nursing.* 29(1):28-35.

Chen, I. J., Yu, S., Wang, T. Z., Cheng, S. P., & Huang, L. H. (2005). Knowledge about osteoporosis and its related factors among public health nurses in Taiwan. *International Osteoporosis Foundation and National Osteoporosis Foundation* 2005. 16:2142-2148.

Dawson, C. (2002). *A Practical Guide to Research Methods: A user-friendly guide to mastering research techniques and projects.* (1st ed.). Cromwell Press: Oxford.

Fain, J. A. (2004). *Reading, Understanding, and Applying Nursing Research: a text and workbook.* (2nd ed.). F. A. Davis: Philadelphia.

Fox, N., Hunn, A., & Mathers, N. (2009). Sampling and Sample Size Calculation. Retrieved from *http://www.rds-eastmidlands.org.uk/resources/doc_download/9-sampling-and-sample-size-calculation.html*

Burns, N., & Grove, K. G. (2005). *The Practice of Nursing Research: Conduct, Critique, and Utilization.* (5th ed.). Elsevier Saunders: Missouri.

Gustavsson, B. (2007). *The Principles of Knowledge Creation: research methods in the social sciences.* (1st ed.). MPG Books Ltd: Cornwall.

Houser, J. (2008). *Nursing Research: Reading, Using, and Creating Evidence.* (1st ed.). Jones and Bartlett: Sundbury.

Hulley, S. B., Cummings, S. R., Browner, W. S., Grady, D. G., & Newman, T. B. (2007). *Designing Clinical Research.* (3rd ed.). Lippincott Williams & Wilkins: Philadelphia.

Macnee, C. L. & McCabe, S. (2008). *Understanding Nursing Research: reading and using research in evidence-based practice.* (2nd ed.). Lippincott Williams & Wilkins: Philadelphia.

McGlynn, E. A. (1998). *Health Information System: design issues and analytic applications.* (1st ed.). RAND: Washington.

Polit, D. F., & Beck, C. T. (2004). *Nursing Research: Principle and Methods.* (7th ed.). Lippincott Williams & Wilkins: Philadelphia.

Robinsoon, S., & Murrells, T. (1998). Getting Started: choice and constraint in obtaining a post after qualifying as a registered mental nurse. *Journal of Nursing Management.* 6:137-146.

Scott, D., & Morrison, M. (2006). *Key Ideas in Educational Research.* (1st ed.). Continuum: New York.

Stommel, M., & Wills, C. (2004). *Clinical Research: Concept and Principles for Advanced Practice Nurses.* (1st ed.). Lippincott Williams & Wilkins: Philadelphia.

Swanson, R. A., & Hilton, E. F. (2005). *Research in Organization: foundations and methods of inquiry.* (1st ed.). Berrett-Koehler: San Francisco.

Tulchinsky, T. H., & Varavikova, E. (2009). *The new public health.* (2nd ed.). Elsevier: Burlington.

Wood, G. L., & Haber, J. (2006). *Nursing Research: Methods and critical appraisal for evidence-based practice.* (6th ed.). Mosby: Missouri.

In: Nursing Research: A Chinese Perspective   ISBN: 978-1-61209-833-3
Editor: Zenobia C. Y. Chan   ©2011 Nova Science Publishers, Inc.

Chapter X

Probability and Non-Probability Sampling in Research

K. K. Yau and Zenobia C. Y. Chan

The Hong Kong Polytechnic University, China

Summary

Research is a way to generate knowledge, theories and validate the existing knowledge and theories to meet need the current needs of heath system (Panacek and Thompson, 2007). A precise and systematic design of sampling is of paramount importance t to ensure the generalizability and representativeness of the population being studied. There are two main types of sampling: probability sampling which includes simple random sampling, systematic sampling, stratified sampling and cluster sampling; and non-probability sampling which includes convenience sampling, snowball sampling, quota sampling and purposing sampling. In this paper, the application, advantages and disadvantages of each type of sampling will be discussed. The importance of selecting sampling strategies, its utilization, effects on the generalizability and representativeness of the studied population are also discussed.

Introduction

The aims of researches are to generate new theories, to find answers and solutions to a specific problems or phenomena; to give interpretations of new facts or observations and to test the existing theories (Panacek and Thompson, 2007). To determine the generalizability and representativeness of the research, the strategy of the sampling is crucial for the success of the research to achieve those goals. Sampling is a process to select a number of samples from the target population to represent the entire population; its purpose is to increase the precision of the research, so that the result can be generalized to the population without studying each one in the population as a whole.; iIn the process, the research needs to clearly specify what population the result may be generalized, the possibility of the repetition of the samples, the selection criteria, presence of bias, the appropriateness of the sample size and respect of the human rights of the samples; it also needs to ensure the efficiency and generalizability of the population of interest by systematic organized, consistent approach and avoid bias (LoBiondo-Wood and Haber, 1998). The sampling includes probability sampling whose goal is to achieve statistical conclusion, validity and generalization of the results to the population; while non-probability sampling's goal is to in-depth and holistically understand the phenomena of interest (Loiselle, 2001). The decision of which sampling methods adopted is dependent d on the objectives of the researches that are set by the researchers. The probability sampling includes: simple random sampling, stratified random sampling, cluster sampling and systematic random sampling; while non-probability sampling includes: convenient sampling, snowball sampling, quota sampling and purposive sampling (Bowling, 1997).

Importance of Sampling in Research

Sampling design can affect the representativeness and generalizability of the research results. The principles of sampling are to avoid biases in the selection and should be economical (Crawford, 1997). Poor sampling may result in sampling bias (Mugo, 2010). The sampling bias means the difference between sample value and population value; there are over-representativeness or under-representativeness when applying the result to the population (Souder, 1992). Kish (1965) states that sampling, which is based on the set rules and operations, is an estimator of the population value and affects the precision of research results. To ensure an appropriate selection of samples, the selection should be comprehensive, for example, some researchers may select the samples from the telephone directory, however, it is argued that the list of population of interest may be incomplete and inaccurate since some subjects may not be included if they are not on the list of the directory; it is also important that every subject has an equal chance of being selected, if the selection is not probabilistic, it will decrease the credibility of the results; it is also true that sampling bias is the result of an inappropriate sampling design (Fowler, 2002). Crawford (1997) states that an incomplete listing of the population and dropout rates are also factors of sampling bias.

Criteria Setting

When the population of interest is defined, sampling criteria will be set; it includes the inclusion criteria which are common characteristics of the sample being selected, such as gender, age, education level, clinical presentations and so on; and exclusion criteria that are the characteristics of elements to be excluded from the research, such as incommunicable individuals who are unable to express their opinions related to the research or illiterate individuals who are unable to complete the self-reporting questionnaires for the researches. Martin (1995) states that population characteristics are is crucial in the sampling design, that means inclusion criteria and exclusion criteria for the selection of the sample fulfills the objectives of the research and exclusion of those not fulfilled should be clearly defined.

Bakitas et. al. stated that to avoid sampling bias, the criteria of selection should be descriptive, clear, objective and understandable.

Sample Size

Kalton (1987) states that sample size is a determinator of the precision of the research, it includes a response rate and non-response rate which is the estimator of the overall population value and costing. There is no fixed rule for the sample size, but it is determined by power level, effect size, significance level and potential attrition rate (Duffy, 2006). The power level means that the probability of the test of null hypothesis is false and produces statistical significance; effect size refers to a family of indices that measures the treatment effect or relationship between the control group and intervention group; significance level (P value) refers the probability of an observed difference between groups is due to chances with a margin of sampling errors (Duff, 2006). The size of the sample should be sufficient during the course of the research to avoid sampling errors (Duffy, 2006). Martin (1995) states that it needs to consider the adequate sample size and its representativeness in the sample selection.

Attrition and Motivation in the Sampling

Bakitas et al. (2006) states that there is potential risk of bias if the non-response rate is high and its representativeness is then affected. The potential attrition rate will also affect the reliability of the results. For example, if 60% of the respondents show that the hypothesis is true while 40% show that it is false, if the attrition is 30% which may all show the hypothesis is false, so the result of the research is completely different.

Souder (1992) suggests that eight motivators for recruiting and retaining the subjects in the research, those are; perception of altruism, effective interpersonal contact, provision of free care, second opinion, reassurance and hope on the subject's medical condition, experience and involvement in the scientific study. Murphy (1993) also suggests that the provision of detailed information about the research, personalized approach, offering of study results, acknowledgement of subject's anonymity and confidentiality are motivators for the participation of the subjects.

Sampling Methods

Probability sampling in which the entire population have ve equal and independent chances of being selected (Sounder, 1992). The sample selected is by randomness, the sampling error by this method can be estimated by an appropriate use of inferential statistics (Woods and Catanzaro, 1988). However, probability sampling has its disadvantages of time-consuming for developing a population list, especially, when the population size is large, thus more resource is needed. Probability sampling includes simple random sampling, systematic random sampling, stratified sampling and cluster sampling (Bowling, 1997).

Simple random sampling is to select the sample unit from a defined population list randomly. Simple random sampling provides an equal chance for every sample, the sampling bias can be minimized and thus increase the representativeness of the research. However, it is time-consuming in terms of developing the sample frame, enumerating the subjects and selecting the sample (Loiselle, 2001). In addition, since the sample is selected randomly, the heterogeneity existing in the selected sample will affect the generalizability of the results (LoBiondo, 1998); the dropout rate is high by this method because the researchers do not know whether the samples selected are accessible. Developing an accurate population list is another disadvantage of this sampling method because some eligible subjects may be inaccessible and out of the list, and affect the generalizability of the result.

Systematic random sampling is to select the sample by a fixed interval (K^{th}) on the population list until the desired number of sample is obtained; it can be presented by a formula "K= N/n" where "K" is the interval, "N" is the size of the population available for study and "n" is the desired sample size (LoBiondo-Wood and Haber, 1998). For example, the study on "Drug compliance of diabetic patients", 200 subjects are needed for the study out of the 1000 population, so K= 1000/200, the interval should be every 5th, that is to take the sample at 5th 10th, 15th ..... on the population list. Systematic sampling is convenient and efficient; however , there is a sampling bias in the form of non-randomness. So it is argued that systematic random sampling is not a true probability sampling because not every subject in the list has an equal chance (Woods and Catanzaro, 1988); and there is some conscious arrangement to develop the population list, especially, the first one on the list that will affect the interval for selection (Crawford, 1997).

Stratified sampling is to divide the population into a number of strata and then to select the sample from every stratum randomly and proportionally or disproportionally according to the population (Crawford, 1997). The first elementary is selected randomly and then having a second elementary selected. In this sampling method, the population data should be available in advance, then selecting a sample from each stratum. Stratified sampling requires the bases of stratification, the characteristics of the population should be used to subdivide the universal population into strata; the sample units within a stratum should be homogenous; the number of strata; its boundaries and sample size within the strata should be considered (Crowford, 1997). This method of sampling can make comparisons among subsets if information on the critical variables have been available, so it can increase the representativeness. However, there is difficulty of obtaining a population list with complete important variable information. Also, it is time consuming and needsed more resources for a large-scale study.

Cluster sampling is to divide the population into a number of clusters and then randomly select a cluster for the study; the principle is from the largest and followed by smaller and smaller units. It also called multi-stage sampling for its successive random sampling (Loiselle, 2001). It is employed when it there is impossible to develop and accurate population list; or it is difficult to randomly select the sample from the list or the geographical distance of samples (Panacek and Thompson, 2007). This sampling method is economical and convenient, but there is risk of sampling bias because the selected sample may not be homogenous (Mugo, 2010).

Non-Probability Sampling

Non-probability sampling means to select the sample by a non-random method, so not every subject in the population has a chance of being selected (Souder, 1992). This sampling method is employed when all subjects in the population cannot be enumerated completely; or it is expensive and inconvenient to include all samples for the study; or some phenomena which are rare or unpredictable (Woods and Catanzaro, 1988), such as a study on comatose patients or HIV patients. The advantages of the non-probability sampling method include: economical, saves time for selection and sufficient subjects for the research; however its disadvantages are the low level of representatives and generalization, potential subjectivity of the researcher (Black, 1999).

The non-probability sampling includes convenience sampling, snowball sampling, quota sampling and purposing sampling (Souder, 1992).

Convenient sampling is to select the most available samples, such as volunteers. It is commonly used to study phenomena seemingly homogenous with respect to the characteristics being studieds (Woods and Catanzaro, 1988). This method is cost-effective and is able to ensure sufficient samples for the research (Black, 1999). Its drawback is a high risk of bias because of self selecting (LoBiondo & Haber, 1998).

Snowball sampling is for the sake of convenience, researchers will select the first subject who will go on to introduce other subjects, such as relatives or friends (Woods and Catanzaro, 1988). It is employed if there is no list or identified population (Black, 1999). This method will increase the sampling bias since there is no way to know whether the sample is representative (Black, 1999).

The quota sampling is employed when the researchers need to ensure adequate representation of a sub-group, the number of samples will be selected until the quota is met (Woods and Catanzaro, 1988). This sampling method can ensure an adequate sample size with appropriate characteristics as the researcher' needs (Black, 1999). However, the result may be over-representativeness or under-representativeness, in addition, there may have many variables or contain an unknown source of bias that affects the external validity (LoBiondo & Haber, 1998).

Purposing sampling is a conscious selection of samples that meets particular criteria set by the researcher, or studying the extreme cases (Russel and Gregory, 2003). It is also adopted when samples with rich and in-depth information are required by the researchers. The researchers will judge which individuals in the population of interest can provide special information or experience for the purpose of the research (Woods, 1988). The representativeness of this method is questioned because the sample is selected consciously by the researcher; the potential subjectivity is present; the data collected may be only specific for the samples selected and are not repetitive to the whole population (Bowling, 1997).

Application pof Probability and Non-Probability Sampling in Research

Probability sampling is commonly adopted in quantitative research which is based on a strong theoretical base and uses numbers to represent reality and discover relationship among variables (Fain, 2009); it is based on the homogeneity and relevant eligibility criteria (Polit & Beck, 2010). Generally, a large size of population with homogeneity is selected randomly to avoid sampling errors (Thompson, 1999) because a large size of population can represent the reality and discover the relationship between variables (Fain, 2009). Non-probability sampling is commonly adopted in qualitative research which aims to obtain rich and in-depth descriptive data to explain the complex phenomena and to generate a hypothesis rather than to generalize the results to a population of interest (Bowling, 1997; Thompson, 1999). Qualitative research is able to discover the meaning of the phenomena rather than to measure the distribution of the attitudes in a population (Bakitas et al., 2006). It can generate validity, meaningfulness and insight to understand phenomena, such as social action, meaning of concept (Panacek and Thompson, 2007). However, Cuchiff and Makenna (2002) criticize that the findings of qualitative research is unable to generalize to the population because it does not use a random sampling approach. Even though there is risk of sampling bias in non-probability sampling in which subjects are not selected randomly, an increase of the sample size can increase the generalizability and statistical power of the research (Pilot & Beck, 2010); on the other hand, the sampling bias can be minimized if the inclusion and exclusion criteria are well-defined for the selection of samples in qualitative research (Panacek and Thompson, 1999). It is obvious that there is great difference between quantitative and qualitative research and the application of probability and non-probability sampling is greatly dependent d on the objective and availability of resources for the research. For a large scale quantitative research, the resource demand should be great for randomly recruiting samples to ensure its generalizability and representativeness; this research may be appropriate for the experienced researcher and ambitious researcher rather than the beginner because they can apply for grant d funding for research more easier. However, if the resource is limited, especially for the research beginner, qualitative research with non-probability sampling may be preferable since the objective of the research is achievable and they can learn the research technique.

Conclusion

Sampling is a process to determine a population of interest, to select a sub-group (target group) and sample for the research. In the process, defining the characteristics of the population according to the purpose of the research should be comprehensive and accessible. The aims of the sampling are to ensure the representativeness, generalizability and precision of the research results. Researchers should conscientiously consider the sampling effects on the validity, effect size and significance of the research. On the other hand, researchers also need to feasibly use the resources. There are probability and non-probability methods. Each sampling method has its advantages and disadvantages on generalizability and representativeness of research results. Probability sampling has advantages of an equal chance for every subject because of random selection, however it is costly and difficult in obtaining a complete and accurate population list; while non-probability sampling is cost-effective because of the selection is controlled by the researcher, however, its representativeness is questioned. Probability sampling is common in quantitative research which has a built-in assumption that there is an objective reality that can be measured in a numeric manner; while non-probability sampling is commonly adopted in qualitative research which needs rich and in-depth descriptive data that can be produce knowledge indirectly and it is not measured by means of quantification (FreshWater & Bishop, 2004).

Author's Background

Yau Ka Kin, a year two student who is studying Master of Nursing in the Hong Kong Polytechnic University.

References

Bakitas, M.A., Lyons, K.D., Dixon, J. and Ahles, T.A. (2006) *Palliative Program effectiveness research: Developing rigor in sampling design, conduct and reporting.* Journal of pain and symptom management 31(3).

Black, T. R. (1999). Doing quantitative research in the social sciences :*An integrated approach to research design, measurement and statistics.* London: Sage.

Bowling, A. (1997). *Research methods in health :Investigating health and health services.* Buckingham; Philadelphia: Open University Press.

Crawford, I. M. (1997). *Marketing research and information systems,* (4th ed.) Center re and Network for Agricultural Marketing Training in Eastern and Southern Africa.

Cutcliffe, J. R., & McKenna, H. P. (2002). When do we know that we know? considering the truth of research findings and the craft of qualitative research. *International Journal of Nursing Studies, 39*(6), 611-618. doi:DOI: 10.1016/S0020-7489(01)00063-3

Duffy, M. E. (2006). Resources for determining or evaluating sample size in quantitative research reports. *Clinical Nurse Specialist. 20*(1)

Fain, J. A. (2009). *Reading, understanding, and applying nursing research* (3rd ed.). Philadelphi: F.A. Davis Co.

Fowler, F. J. (2002). *Survey research methods* (3rd ed.). Thousand Oaks, Calif: Sage Publications.

Freshwater, D., & Bishop, V. (2004). *Nursing research in context :Appreciation, application and professional development.* Basingstoke: Palgrave Macmillan.

Kalton, G. (1987). *Introduction to survey sampling.* Beverly Hills: Sage Publications.

Kish, L. (1965). *Survey sampling.* New York: J. Wiley.

LoBiondo-Wood, G., & Haber, J. (1998). *Nursing research :Methods, critical appraisal, and utilization* (4th ed.). St. Louis: Mosby.

Loiselle, C. G. (2011). *Canadian essentials of nursing research* (3rd ed.). Philadelphia: Wolters Kluwer Health/Lippincott Williams & Wilkins.

Martin, P. A. (1995). Recruitment of research subjects. *Applied Nursing Research, 8*(1), 50-54. doi:DOI: 10.1016/S0897-1897(95)80344-0

Mugo F. W. (2010). *Sampling in research.* Retrieved 24-oct, 2010, from http://www.socialresearchmethods.net/tutorial/Mugo/tutorial.htm

Murphy, C. A. (1993). Increasing the response rates of reluctant professionals to mail surveys. *Applied Nursing Research, 6*(3), 137-141. doi:DOI: 10.1016/S0897-1897(05)80176-4

Panacek, E. A., & Thompson, C. B. (2007). Sampling methods: Selecting your subjects. *Air Medical Journal, 26*(2), 75-78. doi:DOI: 10.1016/j.amj.2007.01.001

Polit, D. F., & Beck, C. T. (2010). Generalization in quantitative and qualitative research: Myths and strategies. *International Journal of Nursing Studies, 47*(11), 1451-1458. doi:DOI: 10.1016/j.ijnurstu.2010.06.004

Russell, C. K., & Gregory, D. M. (2003). Evaluation of qualitative research studies. *Evidence-Based Nursing, April 01*(6), 36-40. doi:10.1136/ebn.6.2.36

Souder, J. E. (1992). The consumer approach to recruitment of elder subjects. *Nursing Research Electronic Resource, 41*(5), 314.

Thompson, C. (1999). If you could just provide me with a sample: Examining sampling in qualitative and quantitative research papers. *Evidence Based Nursing, 2*(3), 68-70.

Woods, N. F., & Catanzaro, M. (Eds.). (1988). *Nursing research: Theory and practice* Mosby: St. Louis.

In: Nursing Research: A Chinese Perspective   ISBN: 978-1-61209-833-3
Editor: Zenobia C. Y. Chan   ©2011 Nova Science Publishers, Inc.

Chapter XI

Data Collection of Quantitative Research Methods

N. Lam and Zenobia C. Y. Chan

The Hong Kong Polytechnic University, China

Summary

This essay notifies the significance of the stage of data collection within the research process. It collects the former theory and the latter practice. The data collected can be classified into two types: quantitative and qualitative. Quantitative data collection is believed to be easier for a fresh researcher. Various quantitative data collection methods are introduced and they are either standardized or non-standardized. The standardized collection methods are well-structured with a high guarantee of reliability. While the non-standardized one, including surveys and questionnaires, measurement scales and biophysiologic measures in nursing research, is more flexible to be adapted to the research approach,. Ttheir strengths are summarized. At last, three important ethical issues should be considered during the collection process.

Introduction

Research plays a significant role in enhancing the quality of peoples' daily life. It helps in developing theory and expanding human's knowledge base. From Grinnell (2001, p.14), he gives research a definition:

"A structured inquiry that utilizes acceptable methodology (i.e. quantitative and qualitative) to solve human problems and creates new knowledge that is generally applicable."

Nursing research is the approach carried out by nurses, usually in clinical settings, by using a systematic process to gain knowledge about improving the quality of patient care.

To carry out a research, a series of stages is needed to be undertaken. This is known as research process. Various approaches (Hek, 1994; Kirk, 1996; Parahoo, 1997; Meadows, 2003) have divided the research process into a different number of stages, but their contents are more or less the same. For a nursing research, the process can be summarized into ten stages (Lacey, 2006). They begin with the developing research question; searching and evaluatingon the literature; planning the methodology and research design; preparing a research proposal; gaining access to the data; sampling; data collection; data analysis; data interpretation; and at the end, implementation of research (Lacey, 2006).

Research is an interactive process where that every stage blends into each other. For example, the stage of data collection links up the former part of theory and the latter part of practice. Once researcher has defined the research question and, related data is are gathered by using a systematic collection method. The selected data is are then analyzed and interpreted to support or argue the original study's hypothesis. In the view of Unrau (2001), the role of data collection is therefore connecting theory and practice throughout the entire research process. Moreover, the data collected can be differentiated into two main types: quantitative and qualitative. They will be described later. Since data collection is such a critical step in the research process, that it will be mainly focused and discussed in this essay, especially for the quantitative one.

This essay consists of four main sections: (a) Differences between qualitative and quantitative data; (b) Various possibilities for collecting quantitative data including standardized measures and non-standardized measures, such as surveys and questionnaires, scales, and biophysiologic measures used in nursing research. This part will be the main focus of this essay; and (c) Ethical issues in collecting data.

As it is mentioned before, data collection is the bridge between theory and practice (Unrau, 2001). It is an important stage which can't be withdrawn from any research. Since there are a large number of methods for gathering data, researchers should determine the appropriate one according to the nature of the problem, approach to the solution, and variables being studied (Fain, 2009). Also, reliability and validity of the methods and instruments applied should be measured to assure the believability of the findings. Before the data gathering measures are discussed, two types of data are introduced.

Differences Between Qualitative and Quantitative Data

There are two types of data: quantitative or qualitative. The former is in the a form of numbers that can make comparisons or test hypothesis, while the latter is in the form of words or pictures for the preliminary investigation of new areas (Fain, 2009; Kreuger & Neuman, 2006). According to Marlow and Boone (2005), people usually wrongly describe the entire research approach by the data collection type used. For a quantitative / positivist research, qualitative data may be collected partly or completely; to the contrary, quantitative data can be involved in a qualitative / interpretist research (Marlow & Boone, 2005). Therefore, it is necessary to clarify that the terms quantitative and qualitative data are referring to the type of data collected rather than the research approach. To be simplified, quantitative data collection is not equal to a quantitative research approach.

As a research beginner, collecting quantitative data is thought to be easier than collecting the qualitative one. It is because objective measurement of a phenomenon is focused during the collection. Quantitative data is are usually collected in mathematical form that promotes analysis in a statistical and scientific way. Also, the large sample size applied has given the support to the believability of data. Oppositely, researchers should have the ability to observe, understand, or interpret the phenomenon so that qualitative data can be obtained. In comparison, the qualitative data method may be more complicated to a fresh researcher.

No matter the qualitative or quantitative data, it is usually involvesd the use of instruments to record or gather data on a particular concept. An instrument can be any equipment, structured interview, or paper-and-pencil test (Fain, 2004). Regarding to quantitative data collection, instruments are used to convert information into numbers so that it is easily used for analysis (Langford, 2001). To choose an appropriate instrument, it is necessary to evaluate its reliability and validity. Reliability, with the meaning similar to consistency, refers to the stability of a result obtained by an instrument. And Polit and Hungler (1997) suggested that the less variation an instrument produces in repeated measurements of an attribute, the higher is its reliability. On the other hand, Vvalidity is the degree to which an instrument measures what it is intended to measure. Criterion, content and construction validity are the three main types to measure the overall validity of an instrument in different dimensions (Bannigan & Watson, 2009). A data collection instrument can be reliable, but without validity. However, an instrument with low validity is usually accompanied with low reliability. Standardized methods, surveys and questionnaires, scales, and biophysical measures in nursing are the common collection instruments found, and they are going to be introduced.

Various Possibilities for Collecting Quantitative Data

Standardized Data Collection Methods

Based on Wilkinson and Mcnell (1996), standardized tests are the tests that have been administered and scored in a standard way. They are the most available and widely used when researchers want to compare results or subjects to a target population. That means the results obtained from a norming sample can be used to represents some populations. Standardized measures have a high guarantee of reliability because they have undergone extensive development, tryouts, revisions, and subsequent administration to a large norming sample (Wilkinson & Mcnell, 1996). Also, they are reviewed periodically. Standardized data collection methods can be seen as the instruments to gather data in a lesser time when comparing with the non-standardized ones. Examples of the standardized measures include the cognitive measures which evaluate how much a person knows e.g. the Differential Aptitude Test (DAT); non-cognitive measures to assess something other than knowledge or skill level; and behavioral checklists which systematize and quantify a subject's behavior e.g. Conner Rating Scale (Conners, 1985).

Non-Standardized Data Collecting Methods

Apart from the standardized data collecting methods, there are non-standardized ways to obtain data. The non-standardized measures have no norming group, the administration and scoring is not done in a standardized fashion (Wilkinson & Mcnell, 1996), they are the instruments developed by the researcher according to the nature of information required. Few examples of the non-standardized quantitative data collections will be described and they are (a) Surveys and questionnaires; (b) Measurement scales; and (c) Biophysiologic measures in nursing research.

a)   Surveys and questionnaires

According to Fain (2004), a survey is a valuable method of collecting data about the respondents' knowledge, attitudes, experience, behavior and etc. Surveys can be basically divided into three main types in nursing research: Descriptive surveys which aim to describe what is existing; Correlational and comparative surveys which investigate and compare the relationship between variables; and longitudinal surveys for monitoring changes over time (McKenna, Hasson & Keeney, 2006).

Questionnaires are is commonly used as tools for of collecting quantitative data for surveys. It collects specific data to answer the research questions defined. It is such a convenient instrument that can be delivered flexibly by hand to individuals or to groups, or through posts and mails across a wide geographical area. And it is less costly compared ing to with the others (Marlow & Boone, 2005). However, relatively low response rates may be one of the shortcomings for this instrument. The expected return rate is just about 30 to 60 percentage (Fain, 2009).

A good construction of a questionnaire can help to collect typical and useful data effectively, so that this process should not be neglected. To design a questionnaire, the types of distribution methods and the respondents invited should be firstly identified since they are the factors to determine questions' nature and language applied. It is better set the topic relevant to the respondents so that a higher response rate can be obtained (Black, 2006). To deal with the question structure, there are close-ended and open-ended questions. Close-ended questions provides a number of choices for answering. It can be picked to receive direct answers and therefore, favor the statistics analysis. Once a variety of answers is required, open-ended questions can be qualified as it allows the respondents to create their own answer (Black, 2006).

b)   Measurement scales

Fain (2009) suggested that measurement scales refer to a set of numerical values which are assigned to responses, and they are available in situations when researchers want to measure the respondents' feeling and thinking of a particular thing. Measurement scales are the instruments frequently applied in collecting quantitative data for measuring a variable. Likert scales and Semantic differential scales are commonly used.

The Likert scale, also called the summative scales, requires the respondents' opinions on statements to indicate which categories they are belonged to, e.g. strongly disagree, disagree, are neutral, agree or strongly agree. A score is assigned for each category. After the summation of the score, the total score is then reflecting the overall degree of agreement with the concept being measured (Langford, 2001). The following is the example of Likert scale shown:

Example 1. Likert scale

	Strongly disagree	Disagree	Neutral	Agree	Strongly agree
This essay is useful	1	2	3	4	5

Another suggested type of measurement scale is Ssemantic differential scales. It is used to measure the respondents' perceptions ives toward a concept by creating a rating measure in between bipolar adjectives such as good / bad, simple / complex. This scale therefore allows an indirect measurement of the respondents' feelings about a concept (Kreuger & Neuman, 2006). Here is the example of a semantic differential scale:

Example 2. Semantic differential scales

How do you feel about this essay?
Good __ __ X __ __ __ __ __ __ __ Bad

Table 1. Brief summary of strengths of various quantitative data collection methods

	Collection methods	Strengths
1.	Standardized measures	• high guarantee of reliability • gather data in a lesser time than non-standardized one • well-constructed
2.	Non-Standardized measures: a. Surveys and questionnaires	• flexible delivery • less costly • effective if well-constructed
	b. Measurement scales	• Versatile and powerful • Simplified measurement of respondents' feeling to something.
	c. Biophysiologic measures	• Favor the nursing research • Objective, accurate, and precise

c) Biophysiologic measures in nursing research

According to Polit and Hungler (1997), Bbiophysiologic measure is usually obtained by nurses or medical researchers in a clinical setting to record patient information. It can be classified into 2 categories. In vivo measures assess the body functions corresponded to some biophysiologic phenomena such as changes in the blood pressure and body temperature. Wwhile for in vitro measures, data is are taken from the extraction of biophysiolgic material from participants and is be subjected to laboratory analysis (Polit & Hungler, 1997). Blood tests areis an example. This measure provides valuable clinical information which favors the easy analysis of quantitative data in nursing research. Also, as a valid and reliable measuring instrument, it has the advantage of being objective, accurate, and precise (Hek, Judd & Moule, 2002).

An appropriate collection method regarding the research problem and the origin's hypothesis is necessary to do a good research. After the brief introduction of various quantitative data collection methods, their application and advantages are known. Above is a table to provide a brief summary of the strengths of various quantitative data collection methods discussed:

Ethical Issues in Collecting Data

At last, after the general introduction of various possibilities for collecting quantitative data, there are three important ethical issues that researchers have to be concerned with during the data collection. Firstly, informed consent should be obtained. All of the respondents should have the right to obtain sufficient information about the research so that they can make decisions on about participating. Secondly, take anonymity and confidentiality into account to protect the identity of respondents. Normally, it is not a usual problem during quantitative data collection since names or contact addresses are seldom requested unless follow-up is necessary (Roe & Webb, 1998). Thirdly, the researchers should avoid any harm to the respondents. For example, protect the respondents with childhood maltreatment from unwanted mental distress. It is the responsibility ties of for the researcher to have a thorough risk versus benefit analysis on the effect of the research on the respondents (Marlow & Boone, 2005).

Conclusion

As a novice researcher, it is important to understand the significance of data collection played in a research process. It is the collection between theory and practice. Although there are quantitative and qualitative data collections, the quantitative one is suggested to a fresh researcher as it simplifies analysis and has a higher believability. No matter what data collection methods are chosen, their reliability and validity should be considered. In this essay, various data collection methods are briefly introduced. For the standardized measures, they are well-structured with periodical reviews so that high reliability is guaranteed, . Wwhile it is more flexible for the non-standardized measures as they are developed by the researcher according to the nature of information required. Three common types of non-standardized measures such as survey and questionnaires, measurement scales and biophysiologic measures are mentioned and their application and strengths are briefly presented. Last but not the least, the researcher should always bear the ethical responsibility during the data collection.

Author's Background

Lam NingNing Lam is, a year two student who is studying Master of Nursing in the Hong Kong Polytechnic University and the Hong Kong Sanatorium Hospital. (Email: ning_1031@hotmail.com)

References

Bannigan, K. & Watson, R. (2009). Reliability and validity in a nutshell. *Journal of Clinical Nursing.* 18, 3237–3243.

Black, T. M. (2006). Using Questionnaires. In Gerrish, K. & Lacey, A (5th ed.) *The Research Process in Nursing (pp.367-382).* UK: Blackwell Publishing Ltd.

Conners, C. K. (1985). *The Conners rating scales: Instruments for the Assessment of Childhood Psychopathology.* Unpublished manuscript, Chlidren's Hospital National Medical Center, Wwashinton, DC.

Fain, J. A. (2004). *Reading, Understanding, and Applying Nursing Research: a text and workbook* (2nd ed.). Philadelphia : F. A. Davis Company.

Fain, J. A. (2009). *Reading, Understanding, and Applying Nursing Research* (3rd ed.). Philadelphia : F. A. Davis Company.

Grinnell, R.M. (2001). Introduction to Research. In Grinnell, R.M. (6th ed.) *Social Work Research and Evaluation: Quantitative and Qualitative Approaches (pp. 1-19).* Belmont, CA: Wadsworth/Thomson Learning.

Hek, G. (1994). The Research Process. *Journal of Community Nursing,* 8(6), 4-6.

Hek, G., Judd, M. & Moule, P. (2002). *Making sense of research: an introduction for health and social care practitioners* (2nd ed.). London: Continuum.

Kirk, K. (1996). Embarking on the research process: a guide. *Health Visitor,* 69(9), 370-372.

Meadow, K. A. (2003). So you want to do research? 1: an overview of the research process. *British Journal of Community Nursing,* 8(8), 369-375.

Kreuger L.W. & Neuman, W. L. (2006). *Social Work Research Methods: Qualitative and Quantitative Approaches: with research navigator.* Boston: Pearson Education.

Lacey, A. (2006). The Research Process. In Gerrish, K. & Lacey, A (5th ed.) *The Research Process in Nursing (pp.16-30).* UK: Blackwell Publishing Ltd.

Langford, R. W. (2001). *Navigating the Maze of Nursing Research.* St. Louis : Mosby.

Marlow, C. R. & Boone, S. (2005). *Research Methods for Generalist Social Work* (4th ed.). Belmont: Thomson Learning.

McKenna, H., Hasson, F. & Keeney, S. (2006). Surveys. In Gerrish, K. & Lacey, A (5th ed.) *The Research Process in Nursing (p.260-273).* UK: Blackwell Publishing Ltd.

Parahoo, K. (1997) *Nursing Research: Principle, Process and Methods.* Basingstoke: Macmillan.

Polit, D. F. & Hungler, B. P. (1997). *Essentials of nursing research: methods, appraisals, and utilization* (4th ed.). Philadelphia: Lippincott.

Roe, B. & Webb, C. (1998). *Research and Development in Clinical Nursing Practice.* London : Whurr Publishers.

Unrau, Y. A. (2001). Selecting a Data Collection Method and Data Source. In Grinnell, R.M. (6th ed.) *Social Work Research and Evaluation: Quantitative and Qualitative Approaches (pp. 1-19)*. Belmont: Thomson Learning.

Wilkinson, W. K. & Mcnell, K. (1996). *Research for the Helping Professions.* USA: Brooks/Cole publishing company.

In: Nursing Research: A Chinese Perspective
Editor: Zenobia C. Y. Chan

ISBN: 978-1-61209-833-3
©2011 Nova Science Publishers, Inc.

Chapter XII

The Uses of Parametric and Non-Parametric Tests in Hypothesis Testing of Nursing Research

Y. C. Kwok and Zenobia C. Y. Chan
The Hong Kong Polytechnic University, China

Summary

Hypothesis testing is the root of scientific research. In quantitative research, statistics are used to accept or reject the null hypothesis in order to answer research questions. In nursing research, statistical tests are often used to analyze the data. There are two main types of statistical tests: parametric and non-parametric tests. The uses and evaluation of these statistical tools are controversial yet necessary. In this paper, differences among parametric and non-parametric tests are depicted, examples and applications in nursing research are illustrated and the evaluation of statistical testing and its interpretation are discussed.

Introduction

In quantitative researches, researchers use statistics as a key tool to compile and interpret data so that their research questions can be answered. Statistics can be grouped into two main types: descriptive and inferential statistics (see figure1). For descriptive statistics, characteristics of the sample, such as the measures of central tendency (mean, mode, and median), standard deviation, variance, and range, will be depicted for describing the variables. No conclusion can be drawn based on these descriptive results. On the other hand, for inferential statistics, it can generalize findings from a sample to a population, which is the larger group from which the sample was drawn. Conclusions about the population will thus be drawn by interpreting the data of a sample. Inferential statistics includes two approaches:

estimation procedures and hypothesis testing (Brase, 2006). Estimation procedures are applied for estimating population value and the accuracy of the estimate. Estimation has two forms: point estimation or interval estimation. Point estimation involves calculating a single statistic to estimate the parameter. Interval estimation involves constructing a confidence interval (CI) around the point estimate. In nursing researches, the hypothesis-testing approach is pre-dominated (Abrams & Scragg, 1996; Polit & Beck, 2004).

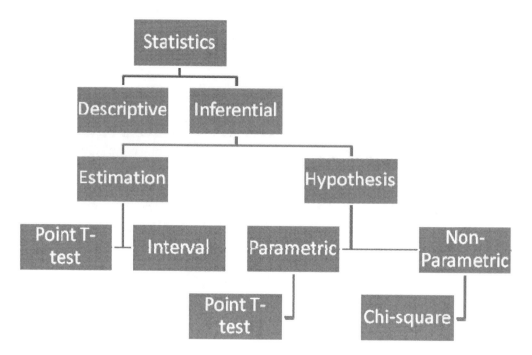

Figure 1. Classifications of statistics.

Hypothesis testing uses sampling distributions and laws of probability to make an objective decision about whether to accept or reject the null hypothesis. The null hypothesis (H_0) is a statement which indicates that there is no relationship between variables, whereas the research hypothesis (H_1) is the statement researchers seek to verify. Several steps are involved in the hypothesis testing. If a test of significance shows that results were statistically significant (not likely caused by chance), then the null hypothesis is rejected. To begin with, researchers need to choose an appropriate statistical test, based on factors such as the level of measurement of the variables. A parametric test concerns the estimation of a parameter, the use of data measured on an interval scale, ratio scale, or higher, and assumptions about the distribution of the variables. T-test and ANOVA are the common parameter tests used in the nursing researches (Boswell & Cannon, 2007). A non-parametric test has fewer restrictive assumptions, and is more likely to be used when the key variables are of nominal or ordinal levels. The Chi-square test is one of the most common non-parametric tests (Urdan, 2005). In this paper, usages and applications of t-tests and chi-square will be illustrated, and the differences among these tests will be discussed.

Parametric and Non-Parametric Tests

In hypothesis testing, parametric and non-parametric tests have s been used for accepting or rejecting the null hypothesis. Parametric tests such as T-tests and ANOVA require assumptions to be met (see tTable1). Basically, those assumptions are normal distribution, data being measured by interval or ratio scale, equal variances when comparing two independent samples (Bowers, House & Owens, 2006). In contrast, non-parametric tests, do not estimate parameters. They are employed when data wasere measured on a nominal or ordinal scale, with no assumptions of normal distributions. Hence, non-parametric tests are sometimes called distribution-free statistics (Polit & Beck, 2004). In general, parametric tests are more powerful than non-parametric tests and are usually preferred (Boswell & Cannon, 2007). Powerfulness can be referred to the likelihood of correctly rejecting a false null hypothesis (i.e. hit). With the same given set of data, a parametric test has a higher chance of correctly rejecting the null hypothesis (more hits), as opposed to a non-parametric test.

Table 1. Assumption comparison between parametric and non-parametric tests

	Parametric	Non-parametric
Distribution	Normal Distribution	Distribution-Free
Type of data	Interval/Ratio	Nominal/Ordinal
Equal variance	Yes	Not necessary
Powerfulness	More Powerful	Less Powerful

There is some disagreement about the use of parametric tests. Some argue that the use of parametric tests should be strictly avoided when the assumption has not been met. On the other hand, many statistical studies have shown that statistical decision- making is not affected even when some of the assumptions have been violated (Armstrong, 1981; Polit & Beck, 2004). The statistical test is described as robust when it provides reasonably valid portrayals of data when some of the test's assumptions are not met during its application (Dunn, 2001). However, in general, when the distribution of a variable is markedly skewed or multi-modal, especially when the model is small or courted as interval level, a non-parametric test is still preferred to the parametric test (Polit, 2010). In this paper, the assumption of the parametric and non-parametric tests is strictly applied since it gives clear guidelines for researchers in nursing to plan their research and analyze the data. To illustrate the uses of these tests, examples and applications of parametric test (t-tests) and non-parametric test (chi-square) will be described in the following sections.

The Uses of T-Tests

In hypothesis testing, t-tests can be used to make inferences about the difference of means between two groups. If the sample means are far enough apart enough, the t-test will give a significant difference. Hence, it allows researchers to make an inference that the two groups do not contain the same mean (Urdan, 2005). It also means that the mean difference is real rather than just random variation. T-tests analyze differences between means on continuous data (e.g. weight, voltage) as opposed to discrete data (e.g. number of children, number of symptoms). They are also particularly useful with samples that have few subjects. T-tests cannot test for differences between more than two groups. In that case, ANOVA should be used instead. In this paper, we will focus on the two-sample test as it is more commonly used in nursing research (Boswell & Cannon, 2007).

There are two types of t-tests for comparing two sample groups, namely the independent samples t-test and the dependent samples t-test. The former t-test is used when comparing the means of two independent samples. The independent variable in a t-test is a variable with two categories. For example, in the quasi-experimental done by de Niet, Tiemens and Hutschemaekers (2009), sleep quality of inpatients in psychiatric wards measured by the Richards-Campbell Sleep Questionnaire (RCSQ) were analyzed by the means of an independent t-test. In this study, inpatients were divided into a treatment group and a comparison group for investigating the effect of music relaxation therapy on sleep quality. The hypothesis of this study was that the assisted-music intervention could improve the sleep quality of the psychiatric inpatients. After data collection, a t-test was used to test the mean score of RCSQ between the treatment group and the control group, because these groups were independent and had no relationship with the experiment result. The experiment was a between-subject design and it illustrated how an independent t-test was applied in nursing research, in which the target group was compared to the control group.

Dependent sample t-test, also called paired t-test, is employed for comparing two means on a single dependent variable. For example, in the study of van Dyck, Lyness, Rohrbaugh and Siegal (2009), a paired t-test was used for analyzing the effect of Vitamin B_{12} supplement on dementia patients with low serum B_{12}. In this study, 28 subjects were selected and their hematologic and metabolic functions were measured before and after 8 weeks of Vitamin B_{12} supplement treatment. The hypothesis being tested was that the post-treatment hematologic and metabolic functions were higher than the pre-treatment level. In this case, the paired t-test was used for comparing the mean differences of hematologic and metabolic functions such as complete blood count, thyroid function studies, and urinalysis. This was a within-subject design, in which the pre-treatment group data needed to match with the post-treatment group data of the same subject. The study design illustrated how the dependent t-test was applied in the nursing research situation that target conditions wereas compared before and after the intervention.

One vital point to notice is that the t-test requires equal sample variance. Harris (1998) suggested that the t-test would provide less valid results if two samples were being compared but had an unequal number of observations in each sample, due to the respective distributions were not all normal in shape, and the sample variances differed from one another by a factor of 10 or more. Hence, it is important for researcher to take note of the sample size of each group, and whether they have equivalent sample size in particular.

The Uses of Chi-Square

The chi-square (X^2) is a non-parametric test used to examine the hypothesis about the proportion of cases that fall into different categories, as when a contingency table has been made. For hypothesis testing, chi-square test of independence or Pearson's chi-square is commonly applied (Urdan, 2005). The chi-square statistic is computed by comparing observed frequencies (which represent the condition we observed in the clinical setting) and expected frequencies (which represent the condition we expected in the world) (Bowers, House & Owens, 2006). The null hypothesis for the chi-square test assumes the absence of a relationship between the independent and dependent variable, that is, they are independent from each other. The Chi-square test can be used for ordinal variables if there are only a few levels (e.g., very low bone density, low bone density and normal bone density). The chi-square test can also be applied to interval or ratio data that hasve been grouped into categories. However, when researchers have numerical (interval or ratio) data, it is often preferable to use the parametric tests with ungrouped raw data as they are more powerful.

In the research of Wangensteen, Johansson, Björkström and Nordström (2010), Pearson's chi-square test was used to find out the critical thinking dispositions among newly graduated nurses in Norway, and the impact of the background data on critical thinking dispositions. California Critical Thinking Dispositions Inventory (CCTDI) was used to measure the critical thinking. Since the subscale scores were not normally distributed, non-parametric tests were used. Chi-square tests were then carried out to test the differences in proportions between groups, i.e., respondents with high vs. low critical thinking scores, in relation to demographic variables measured at a categorical level. In the category of university education prior to nursing, there was a significant difference which indicated that a higher proportion of nurses were found with high critical thinking scores among those with university education prior to nursing education, and those working in community health care. This study displays how chi-square analysis is used (a) when the distribution is not normally skewed, and (b) in the categories.

The Evaluation of the Statistical Tests

In order to evaluate the effectiveness and ultimately, the rigour of the study, several terms are coined for critiquing the use of statistical tests and their interpretation. Operational adequacy is a term for describing the adequacy of information about the data analysis techniques employed in a research paper and appropriateness of the use of techniques for hypothesis testing (Fawcett & Garity, 2009). In order to fulfill the criterion of operational adequacy, the data analysis technique should be clearly identified and described. Selecting the appropriate inferential statistic depends on the theory-testing research design. Data obtained from experimental designs are analyzed using a measure of effect, and data from a specific experimental research design is are analyzed using a specific statistic that is a measure of effect. Another requirement of operational adequacy is appropriate use and whether the results of using the data analysis technique are interpreted correctly. Statistical conclusion validity refers to the correct interpretation of statistical tests of number data (Fawcett & Garity, 2009). This indicates that the researcher can draw the conclusion that the null hypothesis is rejected only if the statistical test is significant at the present level of probability, such as $p<0.05$ or $p<0.01$. The level of statistical significance can be interpreted as the absolute cutoff point for accepting or rejecting a null hypothesis.

In addition, Robinson (2001) and Cohn, Jia and Larson (2009) advocated that criteria for statistical interpretation should include (a) indicating the operational definitions and types of variables in the study, (b) addressing the assumptions of normality, (c) giving an appropriate sample size and reporting a power analysis, (d) providing enough information of the descriptive and inferential statistics, (e) the statistical/analytical approach is appropriate to the level of data, and (f) explaining the differences between clinical and statistical significance. However, not all the research papers can fully satisfy the criteria as listed above. In Hong Kong and Taiwan, only some research papers fulfilled the requirement to provide sample size estimation, for example, "Sample size estimation was based on the assumption that 6.7% of aspirin recipients" (Sung et al., 2010, p.3). Some of the research papers may lack normality testing or reported the results of such testing (Chen, Ueng, Lee, Sun, & Lee, 2010; Lin, Wang, Chung & Liu, 2010; Kang et al., 2010). An example of normality reports is "To check if CCTDI total scores and subscale scores are normally distributed, the Kolmogorov-Smirnov test was performed."(Wangensteen, Johansson, Björkström & Nordström, 2010, p.4). Thus, it is recommended that a formal statistical testing for procedural evaluation programs developed in the nursing field is needed to improve the operational adequacy of nursing research in Hong Kong and Taiwan.

In the study of Cohn, Jia and Larson (2009), 152 quantitative research studies published in the 5 top impact-factor nursing journals were evaluated for statistical methods. The results showed that studies published in high impact-factor nursing journals were statistically sound. However, being statistically sound does not necessarily secure the quality of research paper. Various factors such as quality of subjects and the hypothesis quality can also affect the quality of the research. Moreover, as stated by Hayat (2010), statistical testing is not necessary to represent objective procedures and it does not put away the need for prudent judgment and thought in planning and criticizing a research.

Conclusion

In conclusion, quantitative research uses statistics for testing the hypothesis to validate the questions of the researchers' mind. In hypothesis testing, parametric and non- parametric tests are employed. To analyze the data, parametric tests assume that the distribution of the population is in normal shape; the data is interval or ratio scale and equal variances for independent samples. In contrast, non-parametric tests do not have these stringent assumptions. T-test is one of the most common parametric tests in nursing research. It can be classified into independent and paired t-tests. For independent t-tests, the means of two independent groups are compared. One of the examples in nursing research is the comparison between the treatment group and the control group in a clinical experiment. Furthermore, a paired t-test compares two means on a single dependent variable. One of the examples in nursing is to compare the means of pre-treatment and post-treatment groups. On the other hand, Chi-square is the common non-parametric technique used in nursing research. Chi-square can be applied when testing whether the variables are independent from each other by computing observed and expected frequencies. One of the nursing examples is to test the differences in proportions between groups from different health background.

In order to gain the operational adequacy which indicates the effectiveness of the statistical test shown in the research paper, researchers should fulfill several criteria such as providing enough information of descriptive and inferential statistics, giving an appropriate sample size and reporting a power analysis and addressing the assumptions of normality. In Hong Kong and Taiwan, few researches can fully satisfy the criteria. A formal criticizing model for statistical testing is suggested. Moreover, it is important to note that statistically sounding research findings do not secure the quality of the research paper.

Author's Background

Kwok Yiu Cheung, a year two student who is studying Master of Nursing in the Hong Kong Polytechnic University.

References

Abrams, K., & Scragg, A. (1996). Quantitative methods in nursing research. *Journal of Advanced Nursing, 23*(5), 1008-1015.

Armstrong, G. D. (1981). Parametric statistics and ordinal data: A pervasive misconception. *Nursing Research, 30*(1), 60.

Boswell, C., & Cannon, H. (2007). *Introduction to nursing research: Incorporating Evidence-Based Practice.* Sudbury: Jones and Bartlett Publishers.

Bowers, D., House, A., & Owens, D. (2006). *Understanding clinical papers.* Chichester, England: John Wiley & Sons.

Brase, C. H. (2006). *Understanding Basic Statistics, 4th Edition.* Houghton Mifflin College Div.

Chen, S.H., Ueng, K.C., Lee, S.H., Sun, K.T., & Lee, M.C. (2010). Effect of T'ai Chi Exercise on Biochemical Profiles and Oxidative Stress Indicators in Obese Patients with Type 2 Diabetes. *Journal of Alternative & Complementary Medicine, 16*(11), 1153-1159.

Cohn, E., Jia, H., & Larson, E. (2009). *Evaluation of Statistical Approaches in Quantitative Nursing Research. Clinical Nursing Research, 18*(3), 223-241.

de Niet, G., Tiemens, B., & Hutschemaekers, G. (2010). Can mental healthcare nurses improve sleep quality for inpatients?. *British Journal of Nursing (BJN), 19*(17), 1100-1105.

Dunn, D. (2001). *Statistics and data analysis for the behavioral sciences.* Boston: McGraw Hill Higher Education.

Evaluation of Statistical Approaches in Quantitative Nursing Research 13-*Nurses Response Time to Call Lights and Fall Occurences*

Fawcett, J., & Garity, J. (2009). *Evaluating research for evidence-based nursing practice.* Philadelphia: F.A. Davis.

Harris, M. B. (1998). *Basic statistics for behavioral science research* (2nd ed.). Boston: Allyn and Bacon.

Hayat, M. (2010). Understanding Statistical Significance. *Nursing Research, 59*(3), 219-223. Retrieved from Academic Search Premier database.

Kang, C., Chang, S., Chen, P., Liu, P., Liu, W., Chang, C., et al. (2010). Comparison of family partnership intervention care vs. conventional care in adult patients with poorly-controlled type 2 diabetes in a community hospital: A randomized controlled trial. *International Journal of Nursing Studies, 47*(11), 1363-1373.

Lin, C., Wang, M., Chung, H., & Liu, C. (2010). Effects of Acupuncture-like Transcutaneous Electrical Nerve Stimulation on Children with Asthma. *Journal of Asthma, 47*(10), 1116-1122.

Polit, D. F. (2010). *Statistics and data analysis for nursing research* (2nd ed.). Boston: Pearson.

Polit, D. F., & Beck, C. T. (2004). *Nursing research: Principles and methods.* Philadelphia, Penns: Lippincott Williams & Wilkins.

Robinson, J. H. (2001). Mastering research critique and statistical interpretation: Guidelines and golden rules. *Nurse Educator, 26*, 136-141.

Sung, J., Lau, J., Ching, J., Wu, J., Lee, Y., Chiu, P., et al. (2010). Continuation of Low-Dose Aspirin Therapy in Peptic Ulcer Bleeding. *Annals of Internal Medicine, 152*(1), 1.

Urdan, T. C. (2005). *Statistics in pPlain English.* Mahwah, N.J: Lawrence Erlbaum Association.

van Dyck, C. H., Lyness, J. M., Rohrbaugh, R. M., & Siegal, A. P. (2009). Cognitive and psychiatric effects of vitamin B12 replacement in dementia patients with low serum B12 levels: a nursing home study. *International Psychogeriatrics, 21*(1), 138-147.

Wangensteen, S., Johansson, I., Björkström, M., & Nordström, G. (2010). Critical thinking dispositions among newly graduated nurses. *Journal of Advanced Nursing, 66*(10), 2170-2181.

In: Nursing Research: A Chinese Perspective
Editor: Zenobia C. Y. Chan

ISBN: 978-1-61209-833-3
©2011 Nova Science Publishers, Inc.

Chapter XIII

On Choosing Quantitative Analysis Approaches

Y. H. Lam and Zenobia C. Y. Chan

The Hong Kong Polytechnic University, China

Summary

This essay is a review of the different approaches to quantitative analysis. The aim of this essay is to explain the ideas behind different quantitative analysis methods used in research and through this, explore the differences in the three different approaches, namely, univariate analysis, bivariate analysis and multivariate analysis. With an understanding of these three approaches, a researcher would be able to grasp the distinctiveness of these analyses, the purpose of these analyses and the attainment that these analyses can bring about. Only with a thorough appreciation of these analyses would a researcher be able to plan for the type of methods to use and utilize the quantitative analysis tools well to produce meaningful results. This essay would also include the application of these approaches, in particular the increasingly popular combination of the univariate analysis and multivariate analysis to attempt to explore what these approaches can bring about to the researcher.

Introduction

As a nursing student who has just had a glimpse of what a research is about and how it could be conducted, it seems very important to understand how data should be analyzsed. There are numerous books that talks about the use of statistical data analysis software to analyse the data of quantitative research. It seems to be quite simple to obtain results by just using softwares and clicking a few buttons. However, it is fundamental for any person who wants to conduct quantitative research to understand the basic concepts for analysing data and to have an overview of the different techniques involved to achieve particular goals. With different types of identified variables and the design of the research, different methods should be implemented to analyzse the data (Bernard, 2000; Brockopp & Hastings-Tolsma, 2003). The task of quantitative analysis can be broken down into data preparation, data entry, graphic presentation, data processing and analysis, interpretation of the findings and drawing a conclusion (Sarantakos, 2005). However, not all of these will be discussed in details in this essay. The method of the data analysis is actually pre-determined when drawing a proposal on a research study and what the matter of interested is, therefore this essay would instead focus on discussing the approaches that can be taken in quantitative analysis by first attempting to outline the features of univariate, bivariate and multivariate analysis, and then it would continue discussing how these analyseis could be applied to practice with the exemption of bivariate analysis as the essay would focus more on the use of the combination of univariate and multivariate analysis, which is becoming increasingly popular.

Overview of Different Types of Analysis

Before comparing the differences or identifying the uniqueness of each of the analysis methods, it is crucial to have a brief understanding of what each of the above does and what could be achieved by using one of the analyses as the objectives of analyzsing data is to make sensemeaning of the data. Quantitative data analysis can basically be divided into two forms: descriptive and inferential. The descriptive approach aims to present the data and variables in an understandable way, whereas the inferential approach targets to investigate whether the outcome of the research is a result of the variables or only a chance outcome and to generalize the outcome to include into the larger population (Brockopp & Hastings-Tolsma, 2003). Variables can generally be defined as a set of values that would change with a given problem (Krantz, 2009). However, it does not necessarily need to be numerical since a test variable such as gender can be assigned a quantitative value for research purposes (Trochim, 2000). Variables can be further divided into independent variables and dependent variables. An independent variable could have its own value without restriction and the dependent variable would change with changes in other variables (Dodge, 2003). In other terms, the independent variable is manipulated by the researcher and the dependent variable is affected by the independent variable (Hesse-Biber & Leavy, 2011). The different approaches of quantitative data analysis are determined by how many variables that the researcher is interested in looking into and what the researcher attempts to do. The following table would attempt to identify what a researcher can achieve in using each of the data analysis.

Table 1. The Differences between the different approaches

	Univariate Analysis	Bivariate Analysis	Multivariate Analysis
Variables Involved	One	Two	Many
Purpose	Descriptive	Descriptive/ Exploratory	Exploratory
Analysing	Describing the central tendency, dispersions, frequency distributions, significances	Describing or exploring the correlation or comparison of two variables	Exploring the relationship of several variables or cumulative effect of different variables on another variable

Univariate Analysis

Univariate analysis is the analysis that involves only a single set of variables. Since there is only one set of variables, it is impossible for univariate analysis to explore a cause and effect relationship. The main purpose of using univariate analysis is to describe and summarize a sets of data so as to provide the researcher with the possibility to detect the patterns and tendencies that might be hidden from the mass amount of data collected and thus, it enables the researcher to identify and present some characteristics of a phenomenon (De Vaus, 2002a). Depending on which aspect of the data is to be described, univariate analysis could provide a clearer picture on the set of data by a) identifying the central tendency by calculating the mean, mode and median of the set, b) understanding the dispersion by using range, variance and standard deviation, or c) recognizing the frequency distributions by employing graphs, pie charts and histograms (Bernard, 2000). These would enable the researcher to have a better understanding of the variables which the researcher can then do a better analysis between variables.

Bivariate Analysis

Bivariate analysis, on the other hand, deals with two variables and would enable a researcher to explore the two variables simultaneously. Thus, the main intention of using bivariate analysis is to explore two sets of data to understand their correlations and connections. However, bivariate analysis can be descriptive depending on the research design and hence, Blaikie (2003) depicted bivariate analysis as somewhat on the path between descriptive and explanatory. Fielding (2006) considered bivariate to either illustrate similarities or differences between the variables or to describe the connections or patterns. Brayman and Cramer (2009) provided some similar views that the examination of the connection can take two forms, which it could be either the comparison between the independent and dependent variable by experimenting the extent to which they differ to each other, or the exploration of the relationship between two variables to observe how they might be linked up with one another so that one of the two variables would have a tendency to vary when the other changes in value. Depending on the purpose of the study, different methods could be applied to find out the differences or to explore the relationship. However, it should be noted that most of the time, there is no sharp distinction between the examination of differences and relationship as they are done simultaneously (Langdridge, 2004). Cross-tabulation is one of the most common ways to exhibit whether a relationship is present or not (Ritchey, 2008). This could be done by plotting a contingency table to show the frequency distribution of the two variables where it could be cross-tabulated (Polit & Beck, 2004). Other bivariate methods includinge the binomial test and chi-square test are useful in making comparisons among two variables.

Multivariate Analysis

Multivariate analysis is a more complicated analysis in that involves exploring the link among more than two variables. The major aim of a quantitative research is to establish a causality to prove that 'a variable has an impact upon another' (Brayman & Cramer, 2009, p.8). Multivariate analysis plays an important part to provide an elucidation for such a relationship as it explains the reasons for certain variables happening together to produce an outcome or provides reasons for one variable following another in a sequence of time (DeVaus, 2002b). There are a few methods that could be adopted to facilitate the finding of the relationships between several variables. Multiple regression could be used if the researcher wants to find out the effect of two independent variables on a dependent variable and when the two variables would be likely to affect one another (Everitt, 2010). Other common statistical methods used include factorial analysis and analysis of co-variance

Differences

As Blaike (2003) hasve suggested, the major differences between the three is that in univariate analysis, the main focus is to seek the characteristics of the variable, bivariate analysis makes an effort to search for a pattern, whereas multivariate analysis is to look for an influence. Univariate analysis is descriptive and aims to give significance to a set of numbers, making them logical for the readers to understand. Multivariate analysis is most useful in trying to explain or predict a phenomenon because it can deal with more variables at one time as researchers would often be faced with several variables at the same time when conducting a study but find it impossible to separate them (Polit & Beck, 2004). In summary, using univariate analysis would allow the researcher to understand the data thoroughly as it attempts to study the variable in- depth and systematically. Using bivariate analysis would enable the researcher to understand the relationship between two variables as it involves making associations between the pair and understanding how the association works, while using multivariate analysis would facilitate the researcher to find out the effects of numerous independent variables on a dependent variable simultaneously.

Application of Quantitative Analysis into Practice

After having a brief idea of univariate, bivariate and multivariate analysis, the paper would go further on to discuss the application of the different types of analyses and attempt to see how a researcher would use the different analyses bearing in mind what each of them would achieve and the advantages and disadvantages of using them.

As mentioned before, the type of analysis in which a researcher would use is determined when the researcher submits the research proposal. Therefore, it is crucial that the researcher understands the goal of the research and has a thorough understanding of the tool used. Dempsey and Dempsey (2000) summarized that in choosing the type of analysis method, a researcher should bear in mind that a) they should choose the appropriate statistical methods b) which should be applied correctly in relation to the level of measurements of the data, and

c) the data analyzsed should be in line with the aim of the research and d) that the hypothesis should be tested and the results reported should be accurate. In this instance, the essay would continue to discuss the application of the different analysis with examples extracted from journal articles.

In all types of analyses, the researcher has the responsibility to make sure that the data presented is understandable in the way that the researcher interprets it. Therefore, it is common that tables and graphs are inserted into their research report. For univariate analysis, such tables would include data like the total number of participants, the mean or median values of the groups, the standard deviation or ranges of the groups and may also include p-values, percentages or other descriptive information. A research completed by John, Khan, Mirza, Mayer, Buckels and Bramhall provided a good example ofn this. The team attempted to identify some of the factors that followed re-section in hepatocellular carcinomas and using the univariate analysis, the team was able to identify serum albumin, AFP, re-section margin and recurrence as some of the factors that influenced long-term survival (John, Khan, Mirza, Mayer, Buckels & Bramhall, 2006). This was done by plotting a table that described that data collected showing ranges, mean and p-values.

Univariate analysis is seldom done alone. Brayman and Cramer (2009) pointed out that "the investigation of relationship is an important step in the explanation and consequently contributes to the building of theories about the nature of the phenomena in which we are interested" (p.198). In fact, descriptive and inferential approaches are often used together and usually sequentially with descriptive first and then inferential (Brockopp & Hastings-Tolsma, 2003). In the early stages of a research, using univariate analysis to analyze the data at hands is common. After the researcher has a clearer picture of the variables, conducting a more advanced and complicated bivariate or multivariate analysis would enable an exploration of the relationships between data.

Multivariate analysis can further analyzse the effects of a few independent variables on dependent variables which can be accumulative. In a study by Ling, Kamalarajah, Cole, James and Shaw, the cumulative risk factors contributing to suprachoroidal haemorrhage complicating cataract surgery were investigated by comparing patients from control and experimental groups with a list of significant risk factors that were identified using univariate analysis. Using multivariate analysis, they were able to produce a result showing that patients in experimental groups had 158 times higher risk of haemorrhage if they had the risk factors that were listed (Ling, Kamalarajah, Cole, James & Shaw, 2004). The use of multivariate analysis enables the researcher to explore into relationships and cause and effect of interrelated variables. It is also important to note that the hypothesis confirmed by multivariate analysis may only be true to a certain degree since the analysis is only able to prove that the relationship between two variables is valid to only some members of a sample, but not to the others as a whole (Dugard, Todman & Staines, 2010). In this instance, generalizing the relationship is not possible.

Sarantakos (2005) believed that advancement of technology has brought a number of advantages to quantitative analysis and its procedures like increasing the speed and amount of data that can be processed, lowering the cost to analyzse the data, gaining higher reliability and accuracy and increasing the accessibility of complicated statistics by those not familiar with statistics. With this, quantitative analysis has been made easier for research students to pick up.

Conclusion

This essay examines the different analysis approaches regarding quantitative research. These approaches include univariate analysis, bivairate analysis and multivariate analysis. Univariate analysis can be used to describe a set of data to provide more understanding of it. Bivariate analysis is usually done to explore the correlation of two variables or to do a comparison between them. Multivariate analysis can be done to explore the relationship between a number of variables. The application of univariate in combination with multivariate has also been discussed. There is a limitation to this essay as the author is a student new to this field and has little exposure to conducting research. However, for thate very reason, the author is able to understand the struggles that beginners would have and this essay attempts to answer some of thosee problems that beginners would have.

Author's Background

Lam Yu Hei, Ray is a year two student in the Master of Nursing at the Hong Kong Polytechnic University. He believes that both qualitative and quantitative research can be fun when you understand the tricks to it. (Email: 09691081g@polyu.edu.hk)

References

Bernard, H. R. (2000). *Research methods in anthropology: Qualitative and quantitative approaches.* Thousand Oaks: Sage Publications.

Blaikie, N. (2003). *Analyzing quantitative data: From description to explanation.* London: Sage Publications.

Brayman, A., & Cramer, D. (2009). *Quantitative data analysis with SPSS14, 15 and 16: A guide for social scientist.* Hove: Routledge.

Brockopp, D. Y., & Hastings-Tolsma, M. T. (2003). *Fundamentals of nursing research* (3rd ed.). Sudbury: Jones & Bartlett.

DeVaus, D. A. (2002a). *Analyzing social science data.* London: Sage Publications.

DeVaus, D. A. (2002b). *Surveys in social research* (5th ed.). London: Routledge.

Dempsey, P. A., & Dempsey, A. D. (2000). *Using nursing research: Process, critical evaluation and utilization* (5th ed.). Philadelphia: Lippincott.

Dodge, Y. (2003). *The Oxford Dictionary of Statistical Terms.* Oxford: Oxford University Press.

Dugard, P., Todman, J., & Staines, H. (2010). *Approaching multivariate analysis: A practical introduction* (2nd ed.). Hove: Routledge.

Everitt, B. S. (2010). *Multivariable modeling and multivariate analysis for behavioral sciences.* Boca Raton: CRC Press.

Fielding, J. L. (2006). *Understanding social statistics* (2nd ed.). London: Sage Publications.

Hesse-Biber, S. N., & Leavy, P. (2011). *The practice of quantitative research* (2nd ed.). Los Angeles: Sage.

John, A. R., Khan, S., Mirza, D. F., Mayer, D. A., Buckels J. A. C., & Bramhall, S. R. (2006). Multivariate and univariate analysis of prognostic factors following re-section in HCC: The Birmingham experience. *Digestive Surgery*, 23, 103-109.

Krantz, S. G. (2009). A guide to real variables. Washington, D.C.: *Mathematical Association of America*.

Langdridge, D. (2004). *Introduction to research methods and data analysis in psychology*. Harlow, England: Pearson.

Ling, R., Kamalarajah, S., Cole, M., James, C., & Shaw, S. (2004). *British Journal of Ophthalmology*, 88, 474-477.

Polit, D. F., & Beck, C. T. (2004). *Nursing research: Principles and methods* (7th ed.). Philadelphia: Lippincott Williams & Wilkins.

Ritchey, F. J. (2008). *The statistical imagination: Elementary statistics for social sciences* (2nd ed.). Boston: McGraw-Hill.

Sarantakos, S. (2005). *Social research* (3rd ed.). Basingstoke: Palgrave Macmillan.

Trochim, W. (2000). *The research methods knowledge base* (2nd ed.). Cincinnati, OH: Atomic Dog Publishing.

In: Nursing Research: A Chinese Perspective
Editor: Zenobia C. Y. Chan

ISBN: 978-1-61209-833-3
©2011 Nova Science Publishers, Inc.

Chapter XIV

Validity of Nursing Research

S. M. Tai and Zenobia C. Y. Chan
The Hong Kong Polytechnic University, China

Summary

Validity is important in nursing research since it can be used to determine whether the findings of the research are valid or not. The valid findings are valuable in further research studiesy and nursing development. This paper provides some basic information about validity in quantitative research studiesy including some common types of validity and the threats to external and internal validity. In addition, several methods that are used to establish validity are discussed and the criteria in critiquing validity are also mentioned in this paper.

Introduction

Nursing research plays a significant role in nursing development. For example, it can generate new nursing knowledge for clinical practice (Miracle, 1999), therefore, the care delivereding to the client has ave evidence supporting that it really can promote health to the clients. As a result, the findings of the research , which find out by special measuring instruments chosen by the researcher, are very important (LoBiondo-Wood & Haber, 1998). The performance of these instruments is based on the level of validity and reliability (White & van den Broek, 2004) which should be evaluated that a valid and reliable result can provide a valid conclusion of the research (Avis, 1995). Because of this, the issue of validity and reliability become the main concern of the researchers. Although validity and reliability show equal importance in nursing research, this paper is mainly focuses on validity.

Validity is the extent that the measuring instrument can exactly or actually measure the phenomenon that the researcher is interested in (Treacy & Hyde, 1999). This means that instruments can measure the right thing consistently (Houser, 2008). As a result, the findings that draw from this instrument are more accurate and valid, and the conclusion can be accepted by the audience more easily and can be useful for nursing development.

Different Types of Validity

Validity can be simply distinguished into external and internal validity (Burns, 2000). External validity is mainly focused on generalization (Twycross & Shields, 2004) whichthat refers to the degree that the findings of the research can be applied to other populations (Veerman, Mackenbach & Barendregt, 2007). In addition, the participants who are chosen from the population of interest can be representted the whole population at the time of the study (Roberts, Priest & Traynor, 2006). As a result, results obtained from this instrument can represent the real situation of the whole population.

Internal validity is mainly focused on the extent that the instrument can test the hypothesis and is suitable to the research question (Twycross & Shields, 2004). Actually, there are different types of internal validity, and they can divide into different categories based on the kind of information that the instrument provided and the purpose of the researcher (LoBiondo-Wood & Haber, 1998). This paper only mentions three categories of validity which are content, criterion-oriented, and construct validity (Miyata & Kai, 2009) since they are more common and well-known.

Content Validity

Content validity is whenthat the items of the measurement instrument can represent the domain of content which the researcher wants to measure (LoBiondo-Wood & Haber, 1998). In order to develop an instrument with content validity, the researchers should define the concept and identify the components of this concept first in order to formulateing those related items. Then, they are submitted to a group of experts to assess whether these items are relevant to the concept or not (LoBiondo-Wood & Haber, 1998). Face validity is the subtype of content validity. It is a basic form of validity that the instrument can give some basic idea about concepts of the study (LoBiondo-Wood & Haber, 1998). In order to develop the face validity, the researcher may ask subjects to read the instrument and evaluate the content and whether it seems to reflect the concept that the researcher wants to measure (LoBiondo-Wood & Haber, 1998). Basically, content validity is the rudimentary level of validity in instruments that it simply tests whether the items in the instrument are related to the concepts or not.

Criterion-Oriented Validity

Criterion-oriented validity indicates the degree of correlation between the performance of participants on the instrument and the actual behavior of the participants (LoBiondo-Wood & Haber, 1998). It can be established by comparing the instrument with other similar validated instruments with the same concept (Roberts, Priest & Traynor, 2006). There are two forms of criterion-oriented validity which are concurrent and predictive validity (LoBiondo-Wood & Haber, 1998). Concurrent validity is that the instrument can reflect the actual performance (Houser, 2008). This can be developed by comparing the findings of the new instrument to those findings obtained from an existing valid instrument (Twycross & Shields, 2004). Predictive validity is that the instrument can predict the future behavior or situation (Houser, 2008). These validities y have limitations that both of them are assessed by comparing the finding with other instruments. If there are no existinged instruments for comparison (Roberts, Priest & Traynor, 2006), criterion-oriented validity cannot be assessed.

Construct Validity

Construct validity is the extent that an instrument can really measure the construct which the researcher wants to measure (DeVon et al. 2007). For example, if the researcher wants to use an instrument which has construct validity to measure anxiety, the items in this instrument should measure the concepts which are structurally and also theoretically related to the anxiety exclusively (DeVon et al. 2007). The construct validity can be established by different approaches including hypothesis-testing approach, contrasted-groups approach, and factor analytical approach (LoBiondo-Wood & Haber, 1998). These approaches will be discussed in the next section ofin this paper.

How to Establish Validity in Instrument

In order to establish the validity, the items which may seemn to be related to the research interest are identifiedy first and then different methods are used to assess whether these items are relevant to the concepts and that the instrument developed by these items are really measuringe what the researcher want to measure (White & van den Broek, 2004). In order to have some basic understanding about how to establish validity, the methods used to establish content validity and construct validity are used as an example.

Content Validity

In order to establish the content validity of the instrument, the researchers should define the concept and identify the components of this concept first. Then, based on this concept and also its dimensions, items which are related to them can formulate (LoBiondo-Wood & Haber, 1998). After formulating these items, the content validity of the instrument should be examined by different methods. The most commonly used method is Ccontent validity index (CVI). The instrument is sent to a group of experts and they will evaluate this instrument and rate its items independently by using a Likert-type rating scale to see whether they are relevant to the content domain (Wynd, Schmidt & Schaefer, 2003). For those items with low relevancet levels, they will be modify based on the opinions given by these experts (Yaghmale, 2003) and rated again until all the items are relevant to the domain of content

(LoBiondo-Wood & Haber, 1998). Actually, this method is quite easy to understand and it is widely used in nursing research (Polit, Beck & Owen, 2007),. Hhowever, it has some weaknesses. CVI is mainly focused on whether the items in the instrument areis relevant to the interest of the research, however, it does not measure whether this instrument provides a comprehensive set of items which are sufficient enough to measure the research interest (Polit & Beck, 2006). The other weakness is that the method used to assess the content validity is based on the subjective judgment of these experts (Rourke & Anderson, 2004) which may affect the actual validity of content in this instrument. This can be improved by using other assessing methods to assess content validity of this instrument and by comparing the results of different approaches, the content validity of this instrument can be confirmed.

Construct Validity

In order to establish the construct validity of the new measurement instrument, the items which seem to measure the constructs should be identified first (O'Leary-Kelly & Vokurka, 1998). The construct validity of these items can be evaluated by different approaches including the hypothesis-testing approach, contrasted-groups approach, and factor analytical approach (DeVon et al. 2007) which are commonly used in assessing the construct validity.

Hypothesis-testing approach is based on the theory that the researcher should develop a hypothesis in his research first. If the results of the instrument match the hypothesis, this means that this instrument is construct validity (DeVon et al. 2007). This approach is relatively convenient that no additional assistance is needed, for example, the researcher does not need to invite some experts to assess validity like content validity index.

Contrasted-groups approach uses two sampling groups which are expected to have high and low regions in the measured construct. The scores of these groups, which have significant differences in expected directions, indicate that the instrument is construct validity (DeVon et al. 2007). The sampling groups chosen for this approach should be carefully selected and make sure they really represent the two extreme regions in the measured construct. Otherwise, errors may be occurred in assessing construct validity by this approach.

Factor analytical approach is a statistical method to determine the relationships between different variables. The items in the instrument which are related and belong to the construct are grouped together, and those unrelated items should be eliminated from the instrument (DeVon et al. 2007). Therefore, it is a technique of item reduction (Mendoza et al. 1999) that the number of items in the instrument is diminished and just those related to the construct remain.

There are many different methods to assess validity of the instrument. Since no instrument is absolutely perfect, they both have strengths and weaknesses. Therefore, researchers can choose different methods to assess their instruments and they are recommended to choose those they are familiar with, as a result, the evaluation process of validity is more valid. In addition, in order to provide better valid results of the research, the instrument is usually examined for two or more types of validity For example, the instrument can have both content and construct validity which can assess by using both content validity index and factor analysis. Therefore, the instrument has a higher quality in measuring the phenomena that the researcher wants to measure.

Threats to External and Internal Validity

Although the degree of validity can be successfully assessed by different methods, there are some threats that can affect the validity of the instrument. These threats to external and internal validity can occur at the stages of data collection, data analysis, and also data interpretation during the research process (Onwuegbuzie & Johnson, 2006). Therefore, the researcher should be performed these steps carefully in these steps in order to avoid these threats.

Threats to External Validity

Threats to external validity can limit the degree of generalizations of the research findings (Burns, 2000). It can be caused by different reasons. For example, if the independent variables are not is fail to described clearly by the researcher, it may limit the probability of the future replications of the experimental setting. In addition, the participants may have the Hawthorne effect which means that they know they are in a research study (Burns, 2000).and Aas a result, their responses may be altered and may differed from the real situation. Based on these reasons, the findings drawn from this instrument areis not useful into representing the whole population although it has already assessed its degree of validity.

Threats to Internal Validity

Threats to internal validity can be caused by many reasons including maturation, selection bias and dropout. Maturation is whenthat the participants have a variety way of changes during the experimental period and these changes can cause differences in their responses which are independent to the independent variables (Burns, 2000). Selection bias is whenthat the researcher has bias during the participant's selection for the experimental and/or control groups. This can affect the results of the comparative experiment (Burns, 2000). Dropout means loss of some participants, especially in long term experiments. Since the rest of participants are different from the unbiased sample at the beginning of the experiment, the effect of the independent variables may be affected (Burns, 2000). Based on these factors, the internal validity of the instrument is affected.

After identifying these threats which can affect the validity of the instrument, researchers can try their best to avoid these threats so as to maintain the degree of validity of the instrument.

Critique Validity in the Instrument

As mentioned before, validity of the instrument is very important that it can affect the quality of the findings of the research as well as the conclusions drawn from the findings. In addition, the research is used to find out the reality of the world and also gives explanation to phenomena. As a result, the degree of validity in the research is very important. Therefore, we should have the ability to critique the validity level of the instrument used in the research, when we review a nursing research paper. Here are some basic criteria for critiquing the validity in the instrument.

The assessment of the validity of the instrument should be appropriate and adequate enough to that research (LoBiondo-Wood & Haber, 1998), especially when to those that the researcher used are instruments which wereis developed from others. The design of the research of the current user is not exactly the same as the developer's research. This may affect whether the instrument can successfully meet the goal of researcher or not. As a result, the researcher may need to modify some of items inside the instrument in order to fit his/her goal. Therefore, the reviewer should critique whether the validity of the instrument is appropriate and adequate for this research. In addition, the strengths and weaknesses of the validity of the instrument should be presented in the research paper. Therefore, the reviewer can know the limitations of the findings of the study (LoBiondo-Wood & Haber, 1998) and how to modify the instrument in further studiesy in order to produce a more valid result. Based on these criteria, the validity of the instrument can be critiqued and to make sure the findings are valid enough.

Conclusion

Since validity of the instrument can determine whether the findings of the study are valid or not and it is the main concern in research study, therefore, it is very important in nursing research. In order to provide valid research findings, understanding different types of validity is important in establishing the validity of instruments and several methods which can help to assess validity during establishment are discussed. In addition, the threats that can affect the validity should be identifiedy and therefore they can be avoided in the research. Apart from knowing how to establish the validity, the ability on critiquing the validity of the instrument is also important since that reviewer can justify whether the findings of the research are valid or not. As a result, the findings can be used as an evidence support in nursing research as well as nursing practice and these can help in nursing development.

Author's Background

Tai Shuk Man, with a Bachelor degree of Biology in Hong Kong University of Science and Technology, is a year two student who is studying Master of Nursing in the Hong Kong Polytechnic University. (Email: dindin_christine@hotmail.com)

References

Avis, M. (1995). Valid arguments? A consideration of the concept of validity in establishing the credibility of research findings. *Journal of Advanced Nursing, 22*(6), 1203-1209.

Burns, R. B. (2000). *Introduction to research methods* (4th ed.). London : Sage Publications.

DeVon, H. A., Block, M. E., Moyle-Wright, P., Ernst, D. M., Hayden, S. J., Lazzara, D. J., Savoy, S. M., Kostas-Polston, E. (2007). A psychometric toolbox for testing validity and reliability. *Journal of Nursing Scholarship. 39*(2), 155-164.

Houser, J. (2008). Scientific Inquiry Precision, reliability, and validity: essential elements of measurement in nursing research. *Journal for Specialists in Pediatric Nursing. 13*(4), 297-299.

LoBiondo-Wood, G. & Haber, J. (1998) *Nursing research: methods, critical appraisal, and utilization* (4th ed.). St. Louis : Mosby.

Mendoza, T. R., Wang, X. S., Cleeland, C. S., Morrissey, M., Johnson, B. A., Wendt, J.K. & Huber, S. L. (1999). The Rapid Assessment of Fatigue Severity in Cancer Patients: Use of the Brief Fatigue Inventory. *Cancer. 85*(5), 1186-1196.

Miracle, V. (1999). The importance of nursing research. *Dimensions of Critical Care Nursing. 18*(5), 56-56.

Miyata, H. & Kai, I. (2009). Reconsidering evaluation criteria for scientific adequacy in health care research: an integrative framework of quantitative and qualitative criteria. *International Journal of Qualitative Methods. 8*(1), 64-75.

O'Leary-Kelly, S. W. & Vokurka, R. J. (1998). The empirical assessment of construct validity. *Journal of Operations Management. 16*(4), 387-405.

Onwuegbuzie, A. J. & Johnson, R. B. (2006). The validity issue in mixed research. *Research in the Schools. 13*(1), 48-63.

Polit, D. F. & Beck, C. T. (2006). The Content Validity Index: Are You Sure You Know What's Being Reported? Critique and Recommendations. *Research in Nursing and Health. 29*(5), 489-497.

Polit, D. F., Beck, C. T. & Owen, S. V. (2007). Is the CVI an Acceptable Indicator of Content Validity? Appraisal and Recommendations. *Research in Nursing and Health. 30*(4), 459-467.

Roberts, P., Priest, H. & Traynor, M. (2006). Reliability and validity in research. *Nursing Standard. 20*(44), 41-45.

Rourke, L. & Anderson, T. (2004). Validity in Quantitative Content Analysis. *Educational Technology Research and Development, 25*(1), 5-18.

Treacy, M. P. & Hyde, A. (1999). *Nursing research: design and practice.* Dublin : University College Dublin Press.

Twycross, A. & Shields, L. (2004). Validity and reliability – what's it all about? Part 1 Validity in quantitative studies. *Paediatric Nursing. 16*(9), 28-28.

Veerman, J. L., Mackenbach, J. P. & Barendregt, J. J. (2007). Validity of predictions in health impact assessment. *Journal of Epidemiology and Community Health. 61*(4), 362-366.

White, S. A. & van den Broek, N. R. (2004). Methods for assessing reliability and validity for a measurement tool: a case study and critique using the WHO haemoglobin colour scale. *Statistics in Medicine, 23*(10), 1603-1619.

Wynd, C. A., Schmidt, B. & Schaefer, M. A. (2003). Two quantitative approaches for estimating content validity. *Western Journal of Nursing Research. 25*(5), 508-518.

Yaghmale, F. (2003). Content validity and its estimation. *Journal of Medical Education. 3*(1), 25-27.

In: Nursing Research: A Chinese Perspective
Editor: Zenobia C. Y. Chan

ISBN: 978-1-61209-833-3
©2011 Nova Science Publishers, Inc.

Chapter XV

Is Validity a Must in Quantitative Nursing Research?

Ada K. Y. Wong and Zenobia C. Y. Chan
The Hong Kong Polytechnic University, China

Summary

Quantitative research is a numerical data collection method aimeds at establishing or proving empirical causality between variables. It helps to provide scientific findings for application to the existing clinical problems and for nursing practice improvement. Validity plays an essential role in quantitative research because it ensures the ability of measuring instrument ins reflecting the variables and measuring the concepts of interest accurately. In simple words, validity means the relevance and accuracy of the research. This essay highlights the importance of validity in quantitative nursing research by examining each type of validity, evaluating their purposes and identifying ways to establish them. Choice of validity selection is also discussed, which is made by the researcher basing on the characteristics of target population and measuring instrument, and the availability of a judgmental panel and other comparable validated tools. It is concluded that validity is of high importance in quantitative nursing research. Without establishing validity, the research results generated would possibly be prone to be criticismzed and therefore, spoiling the researcher's effort in conducting it.

Introduction

Research in nursing practice is getting more attention in recent decades. Bassett (2001) mentioned that "with increasing expectations of patients and their families, comes the risk that if the nurse does not provide research-based care, the patient or family is increasingly likely to call the nurse to account" (p.2). People recognize the importance of continuous research activities, as a means for improving nursing care, developing new nursing practice and aiding the evaluation of the nursing process. Quantitative nursing research merits on providing evidence-based numerical statistics reflecteding and supporting the cause-and-effect relationship between variables. It is especially importantce in health care settings because, it helps in tracing back the source of a disease, or to support the effects of newly innovated treatments. In view of this, validity is vital because it helps to build up evidence to ensure the instrument's ability in reflecting the variables and measuring the concepts of interest accurately. In simple words, validity means the relevance and accuracy of the research. Therefore, this essay consists of the following main sections: a) overview of validity; b) types of validity, discussing strategies to establish measuring instrument validity while minimizing the possible threats, and; c) choice of validity.

Overview of Validity

Validity refers to the ability of a selected device to measure what it is supposed to measure in the study (Dempsey, & Dempsey, 2000). For example, if a questionnaire is used to measure the effect of a new nursing practice, then validity is concerneds with about whether the questionnaire is actually measuring that effect or something else. The degree of concept reflecting in the answers collected represents the level of validity of the captioned collection tools. Field & Morse (1985) mentioned that quantitative data research gives an objective nature that enables the researcher to use statistical means to establish validity measurement. For example, results of a closed-ended questionnaire can be analyzed quantitatively and numerically using statistical measures to determine validity.

Without a good research methodology, it is impossible to have good quantitative research. Validity is essential in the evaluation of quantitative research design. As per Cook and Campbell (1979) describe, there are four main quantitative research design considerations:

a) How strong is the evidence that a relationship exists between the independent and dependent variables?
b) If there is a relationship exists, how strong is the evidence that it is the specific independent variable that causes the outcome, and but not the other factors?
c) Can the observed relationships be generalizable across other settings and groups of people?
d) If there are "theoretical constructs" underlying the interested variables, and are these captured in the designs of the quantitative research?

These questions, are, in fact, responding to four aspects of thea validity of a study, they are statistical conclusion validity, internal validity, external validity and construct validity, respectively. They indirectly reveal that quantitative research methodology plays an important role in validity of quantitative research.

Types of Validity

There are three main validity-related issues regarding quantitative nursing research as shown in fFigure 1: a) Validity of the measuring instrument; b) Validity of the research design, and; c) Statistical conclusion validity.

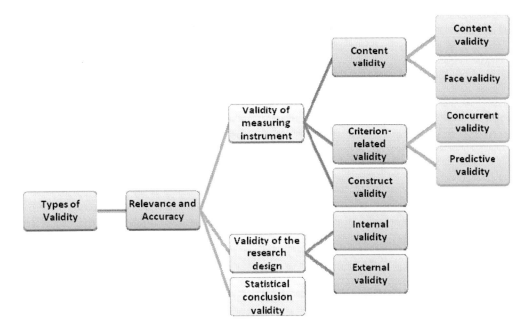

Figure 1. Types of Validity in quantitative research.

Types of Validity

1)   Validity of the Measuring Instrument

When measurement is about translating the reality into numbers, instruments areis a tools or devices that helps to measure a concept. Validity of the measuring instrument is concerned withs about the selection of instruments that is able to reflect the concept of interests truly through data collection. There are three main approaches in assessing the validity of the instrument of quantitative research, they are: Content Validity, Criterion-Related Validity and Construct Validity.

a)   Content Validity

Content validity is concerneds with about whether the instrument is able to measure the concept with adequate coverage. As Roberts and Burke (1989) mentioned, this approach is usually used in the development of questionnaires or interview guides. According to Roberts & Burke (1989), the fundamental of content validity lies in expert judgment and validation from literature review. There are two common ways in establishing content validity: i) Critical literature review. Brink and Wood (1994) describe a method in forming content validity is to make comparisons, between the measurement content with known literature on the selected topic. It aims at evaluating whether the tool represents the literature accurately; ii) Use of judge panels. Referring to Brink and Wood (1994), "use of experts" means calling up a group of people who are knowledgeable about the content of the research topic, then asking them to make judgments on the instrument to see whether it appears to be workable and adequately covers the content that the researchers want to cover.

Some people may be confused about content validity and face validity. Fitzpatrick (1999) describes face validity ias an unscientific way of evaluating an instrument to see if it looks sound and fit for the research, such as asking friends or self to look over the instrument and seethink if it makes sense, but these people may lack knowledge about the area and therefore, the advice maybe superficial and miss out on some important issues.

In my opinion, if content validity has not been addressed, the result generated may become out of focus and fails to address the core concerns of the research question. Therefore, when formulating the tools of measurement, such as a questionnaire, try to do it after reviewing literatures on the selected topic to ensure the questions constructed haves adequate coverage on the content of interest. "Use of experts" is good to use in clinical surveys, especially for newly developed measuring tools, or a modified tool from an existing instrument, by asking doctors or specialty nurses who haveget expert knowledge on the interest area to evaluate the coverage and adequacy of the content of the measuring tool.

b)   Criterion Validity

Criterion validity addresses on making valid comparisons with a criterion, such as comparing the results generated by a validated instrument with the original tools concurrently, or with a future phenomenon to see whether the original tools predict correctly. According to Roberts and Burke (1989), "Determining criterion validity involves comparing the results obtained through the use of an instrument with a particular population sample to the results of some criterion measure believed to be valid for that population"(p.253). Criterion validity evaluation can be classified into two main categories: i) Criterion-Concurrent validity. It means comparing the result with an established instrument for the same target populations to see its validity. If the two results are highly co-related, it indicates that there is a concurrent validity for test; ii) Criterion-Predictive validity. It aims at measuring the predictability of the measuring instrument to some future occurrence accurately, which can be achieved by adapting the longitudinal research approach, measuring the variables of interest now and then follow the sample of people over a period of time to see if the event occurs as predicted.

In clinical research settings, I think concurrent validity is best used for improving the existing measuring tools, therefore, it is able to generate a research result that is better capturesd the current traits or phenomenon. As one of the difficultiesy in achieving criterion validity, as per Roberts and Burke (1989) mentioned, is to find a criterion instrument that has already been validated with a similar research population. But, if it is used for existing tools improvement for better captured concepts captured, the difficulty can be justified. Concurrent validity can also be used in nursing research as the disease is a life-long process in nature, a longitudinal approach is applicable, especially those long-term inpatient. But one may also have to consider for the ethical issue.

c)   Construct Validity

Construct validity refers to the extent to which an instrument or test measures an intended hypothetical concept or construct. As Roberts and Burke (1989) mention, construct validity aims at examining how well the researcher has translated the abstract concepts of interest from the research problem into valid measures on the research instrument. According to Brink & Wood (1994), construct validity is useful for measuring traits and feelings such as generosity, grief and satisfaction. Therefore, are two common approaches are involved in establishing construct validity: i) The known group method: It involves comparing the result between two groups, for which there is a likely observable different; ii) The Multi-trait, - multi-method matrix approach developed by Campbell and Fiske (1959). It involves using the concepts of convergence and discrimination. Convergence means that an instrument constructed is able to yield a similar result with other known concept- measuring instruments with the same subjects, while discrimination means an instrument is able to generate a different result with those using other instruments to test for a slightly different but related concept on the same group of people.

In my opinion, a limitation of construct validity is that it is very time-consuming in requiring a number of instruments / groups to make a measuring comparison. Careful and accurate statistical analysis is required in performing this type of validity establishment because any data collection error may spoil the result generated and provide a faulty instrument validity conclusion.

2)   Validity of the research design

The two validities relating to research design are the Internal and External validity.

a)   Internal validity

It focuses on whether the independent variable actually makes a differencet. Its is concerned with is about whether there is any other possible explanation to the causal relationship generated from the instrument. Minimizing the influence of extraneous variables is one of the methods in attaining internal validity. Lusardi and Fain (2001) said the use of control groups and randomizations are able to reduce the impacts or threats posted by extraneous variables.

b)   External validity

It focuses on the degree of measuring results that is able to generalize to the larger population. It is concernd withis about the representativeness of the sample. External validity can be achieved through the use of randomization. According to Brink & Wood (1994), random sampling is intended to produce a representative sample, providing that the sample size is large enough to include all of the relevant extraneous variables.

I think the key elements addressed in the internal and external validities are the issue of control over extraneous variables and the degree to which the sample represents the population representatively.

3) Validity of the statistical conclusion

Statistical conclusion validity concerns the strength of evidence that there is an empirical relationship exists between two variables, which is, the first step in establishing. In simple words, establishing statistical conclusion validity means making valid statistical ratiocination. There are two aspects concerning its establishment: i) Statistical power. It refers to the ability of the research to detect true relationships among variables. The use of a large sample is one of the ways to achieve sufficient statistical power. Sometimes when the sample is too small, the analysis may fail to reflect the relationship between the independent and dependent variables, hence, leading to low statistical power; ii) Maximize group differences to enhance statistical conclusion validity. It aims at maximizing their differences on the dependent variable. Sometimes when the independent variables, such as the therapeutic treatments provided to patients, are not very different, the statistical analysis might not be sensitive enough to detect its existence.

Table 1. Examples of quantitative research and types of validity chosen

Studies	Purpose	Duration	Settings	Samples	Choice of validity
McInerney, 2008	Measure the effect of multiple strategies in reducing hospital-acquired prevalence rate	Every 6 months for 4.5 years while multiple strategies were implemented	548-bed, 2-shopital systems in Southwest Florida	All adult patients with the exception of those admitted for obstetric or mental health care	Large sample size used, which enhances the statistical power of the statistical conclusion validity Longitudinal approach adapted to see the effect of preventive measures overtime, which addresses the criterion-predictive validity
Frost, & Daly, 2010	To explore GP's attitudes to nurse-led initiatives in the care of children with asthma	2005 to 2007	In the four PCTs of a large cosmopolitan English Midlands city	All GPs registered in the city boundary (n=541), respond rate is 43.6 percent, 236 responded	A 17-item questionnaire was developed from the literature, professional experience and the local context, which addressesing the content validity

Choice of Validity

Wood and Haber (1998) mentioned that, "the choice of a validation method is important and is made by the researcher on the basis of the characteristics of the measurement device in question and its utilization" (p.348). Below is a table showing the two examples of quantitative research and the type of validity chosen.

Conclusion

This essay highlights the importance of validity in quantitative nursing research, examines each type of validity and evaluates their purpose. The Rresearcher has to consider the question of validity early in the research process, such as literature review and methodology stages. Adequate literature reviews on the topic helps constructing meaningful measuring instruments and assists in establishing the content validity. For the methodology, it is the sampling and method of measurement parts that helps aiding validity. A representative sample gives external validity as its result can be generalized to the target population. The use of randomization helps to reduce the impacts of extraneous variables to the result hence, achieving internal validity. A Llarger sampling size gives a greater statistical power enhancing the statistical conclusion validity. Other types of validity are concerneds withvery much about the measuring instrument, researcher can ensureing the validity of the instrument by using an existing, well-tested tool, modifying a pre-existing one to suit local conditions, or to develop a new instrument with validating. If a new instrument is developed, different validity tests should be carried out to ensure its measuring ability, such as using judge panels to judge the appropriateness of a questionnaire, comparing the test result with other well-established instruments for the same target population and see if there is a highly correlated result (convergence) generated when testing on the same concept, or a different result (discrimination) when testing on a slightly different but related concept. In conclusion, without establishing validity of a research, the founfindings generated would be possibly prone to be criticized by others and ruining the researcher's effort in conducting the research.

Author's Background

Wong Ka Yi, Ada, a year two Year 2 student of who is studying Master of Nursing, The Hong Kong Polytechnic University. (Email: mn_wky@hotmail.com)
Ka Yi Wong, (Email: mn_wky@hotmail.com)

References

Anthony, D. (1999). *Understanding advanced statistics: a guide for nurses and health care researchers*. London: Churchill Livingstone. (Anthony, 1999).

Bassett, C. (2001). *Implementing research in the clinical setting.* London and Philadelphia: Whurr Publishers.

Brink, P. J., & Wood, M. J. (1994). *Basic steps in planning nursing research: from question to proposal.* London: Jones and Bartlett Publishers.

Cook, T.D., & Campbell, D.T. (1979). *Quasi-experimental design and analysis issues for field settings.* Chicago: Rand McNally.

Dempsey, P. A., & Dempsey, A. D. (2000). *Using nursing research: process, critical evaluation, and utilization,* 5th edition. New York: Lippincott.

Fain, J. A. (2001). Principles of Measurement. In James A. Fain (Ed.), *Reading, understanding, and applying nursing research: a text and workbook* second edition (pp. 107-123). Philadelphia: F.A. Davis Co.

Ferguson, L.(2004). External validity, generalizability, and knowledge utilization. *Journal of nursing scholarship,* 36, 16-22.

Fitzpatrick, J. J. (1999). *Nursing research digest.* New York: Springer Publishing Company.

Frost, S., & Daly, W. (2010). Nurse-led asthma services for children and young people: a survey of gps' views. *Paediatric Nursing,* 22(8), 32-36.

Hopkins, W. G. (2000). Quantitative research design. Sportscience, 4(1), Retrieved from *http://www.garnetthenley.com/ResDesign/DesignTypes.pdf.*

Knapp, T. R. (1985). Validity, reliability, and neither. In Downs F.S. (Ed.), *Readings in research methodology* (pp. 223-227). Lippincott.

Loiselle, C. G., McGrath, J. P., Polit, D. F., & Beck, C. T. (2007). *Canadian essentials of nursing research,* second edition. Lippincott Williams & Wilkins.

Lusardi, P. T., & Fain, J. A. (2001). Selecting a quantitative research design. In James A. Fain (Ed.), *Reading, understanding, and applying nursing research: a text and workbook,* second edition (pp. 173-200). Philadelphia: F.A. Davis Co.

McInerney, J. A. (2008). Reducing hospital-acquired pressure ulcer prevalence through a focused prevention program. *Advances in skin & wound care,* 21(2), 75-78.

Roberts, C. A, & Burke, S. O. (1989). *Nursing research: a quantitative and qualitative approach.* Boston: Jones and Bartlett publishers.

Polit, D.F., & Hungler, B. P. (1989). *Essentials of nursing research: methods, appraisal, and utilization,* second edition. Philadelphia: Lippincott.

Wood, G. L., & Haber, J. (1998). *Nursing research: methods, critical appraisal, and utilization,* fourth edition. Mosby.

In: Nursing Research: A Chinese Perspective
Editor: Zenobia C. Y. Chan

ISBN: 978-1-61209-833-3
©2011 Nova Science Publishers, Inc.

Chapter XVI

Understanding Reliability in Quantitative Nursing Research

S. P. Lam and Zenobia C. Y. Chan

The Hong Kong Polytechnic University, China

Summary

In clinical settings, it is commonly using quantitative approach in conducting nursing research is commonly used. Ssince it is a simpler, faster, more feasible, objective and systematic way to generate data with a goal to obtain findings that help to evaluate the current nursing interventions and enhances better nursing care in the clinical system. Different data collection instruments are used in this type of research. The degree of reliability and validity of the instruments are the two essential issues in ensuring the degree of accuracy of the outcome. This paper will mainly focus on one of the issues – "Reliability". An overview of the quantitative nursing research is first provided, and "Reliability" is defined. Then, a discussion in related to the importance of testing reliability is given. Finally, two commonly used examples of reliability tests: test– retest reliability and interrater reliability are provided.

Overview of Quantitative Nursing Research

As stated by Fitzpatrick (1999), much of the history of nursing research involved quantitative research. Properly applied quantitative nursing research can advance the scientific basis of nursing as well as provide a potent tool for defining and evaluating the outcomes of nursing care. Nowadays, quantitative research plays an increasingly valuable role in nursing studies to determine the efficacy of nursing interventions through providing required measurements and needed indicators.

Quantitative research consists of the collection, tabulation, summarization, and analysis of numerical data (Fitzpatrick, 1999). It involves quantifying concepts or variables by using different instruments in different data collection methods such as structured interviews, questionnaires and observations. Quantitative research is actually developed from a strong theoretical base, and using a structured design to determining the true relationship between independent and dependent variables with an outcome orientation. It also focuses on an approach that emphasizes measuring and explaining variables, verification of data, testing of theoretical relationships, and prediction of events. Therefore, in this type of research, the two important characteristics are measurement and testing. As a result, within quantitative research, statistical significance, validity and reliability are vital factors for producing a trustworthy outcome in nursing research.

Reliability in Quantitative Research

In quantitative research, it involves measurement which is the systematic process of assigning numerical values to concepts and reflects properties of those concepts. Besides, it also uses a variety of instruments to define each variable being considered and to give meaning to the data collected. In quantitative nursing research, many commonly used instruments are questionnaires, observations and rating scales. Actually, the characteristics of measuring instruments are essential to determine the meaning of the collected data and the degree of accuracy of the resulting findings (Fain, 2009). However, each kind of instrument involves measurement error. In order to provide data that is are more accurately a reflection of the truth, each of the researchers has to attempt to reduce the measurement errors. To achieve the goal, the most important issues to consider are the reliability and validity of the instrument used in collecting data. In this research essay, it only focuses on the introduction of "Reliability" and discusses how the reliability tests help to determine the degree of measurement error and the significance of the research outcome.

"Reliability" is one of the characteristics of the instrument in measurement. To define "Reliability", we may ask how a measurement scale works consistently or dependably in measuring what it is supposed to be measureding (Polit & Hungler, 1995). In other words, it is concerned and tested when assessing the accuracy of a measuring instrument. Generally, "reliability" in quantitative research can be referred to or classified into three forms that include stability, internal consistency and equivalence of the measurement scale.

Stability is the reproducibility of responses over time of a systematic pattern. OIn the other words, it is the extent to which the same results are obtained on repeated administrations of the instrument (Bannigan, & Watson, 2009). It measures the consistency of the responses on an instrument. It is commonly measured by the test-retest approach. The problem associated with stability is that it is unreasonable to assume that the concept remains unchanged over time.

Internal consistency is used to reveal how well the different items measure the same characteristic (Bannigan, & Watson, 2009). From this perspective, reliability is defined as consistency across items of an instrument, with individual items being individual questions. Therefore, it is not applied to a single items, but groups of items that are thought to measure different aspects of the same concept. For example, in order to measure the depression level, different questions (items) are designed. Each question implies a response with 5 possible values on a Likert scale, e.g. scores 0, 1, 2, 3, 4, 5. Responses from a group of respondents have been obtained. In reality, answers to different questions vary for each particular respondent, although the items are intended to measure the same aspect or quantity. Therefore, the smaller the variability, the greater the internal consistency reliability of the survey instrument is. The internal consistency can be measured with a different approach, for examples, split-half technique and Cronbach's alpha. Unlike the stability, internal consistency isdoes not concerned with about fluctuation over time.

Equivalence is the consistency of responses across a set of items so that there is evidence of a systemic pattern (Fitzpatrick, 1999)). Since responses toward the items can be affected and varied by different external factors, such as the language and the manner that the researcher used. It can be addressed in two ways; that is the use of the scale by the same administrators at the same time or administering two parallel forms of the same scales to the same sample successively. Therefore, the inter-rater approach and alternative form approach can be use to evaluate the equivalence of the instrument of the measurement.

Since the researcher has classifiedy the reliability into different forms, a variety of reliability tests are developed to assess the degree of reliability in response to the classification and needs. Following, it gives an explanation related to the needs for conducting reliability tests in quantitative research.

The Needs for Conducting Reliability Tests

There are two reasons for conducting reliability tests. The first reason is that .the reliability provides a measure of the extent to which the instrument for data collection reflects random measurement errors. One the other hand, some studiesy stated that "the less variation an instrument produces in repeated measurements of an attribute, the higher its reliability" (Polit & Hungler, 1995) . Ssince, there will always be a degree of measuring error. The measurement error is actually made up of random and systemic components. Maximizing the instrument's reliability helps to reduce the degree of random errors associated with the measurement. Errors due to response differences results from distracting the respondent, the state or mood of the respondent, the way questions are asked are examples of random errors. Therefore, in order to gain a reliable data in the research, we need to measure the degree of reliability of the measuring tool. Besides, bywith the understanding the correct method in measuring the reliability, we can correctly evaluate and justify the degree of worthiness of the data during the literature review.

Another reason is that a reliability test is a precursor to test validity. Reliability is said to be a pre-requisite for validity as there is little chance of measuring what we say we are measuring if we cannot measure it consistently (Holm & Llewellyn, 1986). That is, if the measurement scale cannot be assigned consistently, it is impossible to conclude that the result obtained is accurately measuring the area of interest. Validity refers to the extent to which a scale measures what it is intended to measure. For example, it is necessary to consider whether the patient understands the question being asked or not during clinical research.? However, the process of formally assessing the validity of a measurement can be quite complicated and time-consuming. Therefore, it is viewed that the process of testing validation is often begins with reliability analysis. If the test is unreliable, it is time-wasting in investigating whether it is valid or not as it will not be.

With an the understanding about the need for measuring the reliability, the coming part will introduce two commonly used reliability tests, and the issue that concerned when they are used by researcher.

Test-Retest

The test-retest method is a commonly used way of testing the stability of an instrument over time. In this method, two identical measuring instruments/tests are given to the same group of individuals at two different times, and then the scores are compared. The extent that two scores are consistent over time is referred to as the coefficient of stability. Test-retest uses a statistical procedures to elucidate a coefficient of stability (reliability coefficient), the range of the coefficient is from zero to one. A completely reliable test has a reliability coefficient of one, and a completely unreliable test has a reliability coefficient of zero. Therefore, the higher the coefficient, the more stable the measure (Polit & Hungler, 1995). Some researchers suggested that stability indexes are most appropriate for relatively enduring characteristics such as personality, abilities, or certain physical attributes such as height (Bannigan & Watson, 2009). Perfection is impossible. There is no test that will yield entirely the same results from test to test, so it is necessary to determine what an acceptable level of error is. Most researchers accept a lower level, 0.7, 0.8 or 0.9, depending upon the particular field of research.

In the test-retest method, the amount of time that elapses between the two testing is a concern. Some researchers suggested that the administrations were best separated by a two to four week period (Holm & Llewellyn, 1986). However, others argued that there was no methodological justification for greater than a two-week time interval, the time interval may actually be as brief as one day or as long as one year. With a short time interval, usually no longer than four weeks, the test-retest gives a higher coefficient of stability. However, if the interval is too short, memory of the responses given during the first test may influence responses during the second test. Even if a test-retest process is applied with no sign of intervening factors, there will always be some degree of error. There is a strong chance that subjects will remember some of the questions from the previous test and perform better. As a result, it leads to overestimatinge of stability due to memory (Fain, 2009) Therefore, when we are reading research reports, we have to be cautiouson in regarding how stable the measurement is when researchers do not indicate the length of time between the two testing.

The second problem is that it is impossible to remove confounding factors completely. Confounding factors are variables that the researcher failed to control or eliminate, and can lead to damage of the internal validity of an experiment or measurement. It can adversely give negative influence to the relationship between the independent and dependent variables. As a result, this may cause the researcher to analyze the results incorrectly. The example of a confounding factor is that subjects may actually change as a result of the first test administrations, such as attitude can be changed, fear or anxiety can be developed and altered by the passage of time, particularly with a long time interval between testing situations, it may affect the individuals performance in the two tests, and lead to a variance of the results. Researchers must anticipate and address the potential confounding factor during the research design to maintain high stability of the measurement. To decrease the chances of a few subjects skewing the results, the test for reliability is much more accurate with large subject groups, drowning out the extremes and providing a more accurate result.

Interrater

Apart from test-retest reliability, interrater reliability will be examined. It is a reliability test that measures the index of the equivalence and consistency between scorers (raters). In some studies, researchers collect data by having raters evaluate a particular situation. It may be expressed in terms of a correlation coefficient between the scores assigned to the observed behaviors by two or more observers or in terms of a percentage of agreement between scorers.

Determining interrater reliability is very common in nursing research and is used in many observational studies. One popular statistical procedure that quantifies the degree of consistency among raters is called Cohen's Kkappa. This statistical procedure is used with nominal data and is designed for situations in which raters classify the items being rated according to discreet categories. If all raters agree that a particular item belongs in a given category, and there is total agreement for all items being evaluated, then Cohen's kappa assumes the value of 1.0 to the extent that raters disagree, Cohen's kappa value becomes smaller.

In this type of reliability test, the main concern is the potential problem that results from the effect of the observers' or scorers' own attitudes and perceptions on their evaluations of the data collected. To decrease the limitation mentioned above, interrater reliability can be strengthened by establishing clear guidelines and through experience. If a clear and concise instructions about how to rate or estimate behavior is given to the observers, the interrater reliability will properly be increases. One the other hand, researchers who have worked together for a long time will be fully aware of each other's strengths, and will be surprisingly similar in their observations, therefore, their experience also contributes to the increasing the interrater reliability.

Conclusion

In conclusion, quantitative approach is widely and commonly used in nursing research. Quantitative nursing research is an objective and systematic process that involves quantifying concepts or variables by using different instruments. In this type of research, measurement and testing are prominent characteristics. We emphasis that reliability is one of the characteristics of the measuring instrument that affects the accuracy of the finding produced. The Ddefinition of reliability was provideds and it is actually included in three types: stability, internal consistency and equivalence. Different tests are used to test different types of reliability of the instrument. This essay introduces two commonly used reliability tests in quantitative nursing research, and examines some concern when using them in clinical settings. It is essential and beneficial for the novice researcher to understand the importance of reliability tests to research. B because it helps them to maximize the consistency of the instrument used in data collection and thus, the accuracy of the finding. Besides, it also helps them to justify whether the instrument used by other researchers is appropriate enough and the finding is trustworthy to read during literature review.

Author's Backgound

Lam Siu Ping, Pinky, a year two student who is studying Master of Nursing in the Hong Kong Polytechnic University and the Hong Kong Sanatorium Hospital. (Email: Pinkylam_926@hotmail.com)

References

Alderman, A.K., & Salem, B. (2010). Survey research. *Plastic & Reconstructive Surgery. 126*(4), 1381-1389.

Angst, F., Goldhahn, J., Pap, G., Mannion, A. F., Roach, K. E., Siebertz, D., Drerup, S.Schwyzer, H. K., & Simmen, B. R. (2007). Cross-cultural adaptation, reliability and validity of the german shoulder pain and disability index (SPADI). *Rheumatology (Oxford)*, *46*(1), 87-92.

Bannigan K., & Watson R. (2009). Methodological paper: reliability and validity in a nutshell. *Journal of Clinical Nursing*, *18*(23), 3237-3243.

Burns, N., & Grove, S.K. (2001). *The Practice of Nursing Research: Conduct, Critique, and Utrilization*, (4th ed.). Philadelphia: W.B. Saunders Company.

Clemons, J. M., Campbell, B., & Jeansonne, C. (2010). Validity and reliability of a new test of upper body power. *Journal of Strength & Conditioning Research,24*(6), 1599-1565.

Fain, J.A. (2009). *Reading, understanding, and applying nursing research* (3rd ed.). Philadelphia: F.A. Davis Co.

Fitzner, K. (2007). Reliability and validity: a quick review. *Diabetes Educator*, *33*(5), 775-780.

Fitzpatrick, J.J. (1999). *Nursing Research Digest*. New York: Springer Publishing Company.

Freshwater, D., & Bishop, V. (2004). *Nursing Research in Context: Appreciation, application and professional development*. Houndmills: Palgrave Macmillan.

Holm, K., & Llewellyn, J.G. (1986). *Nursing Research for Nursing Practice*. Philadelphia: W.B. Saunders Company.

LoBiondo-Wood, G., & Haber, J. (1986). *Nursing Research: Methods, Critical Appraisal, and Utilization*. Toronto: The C. V. Mosby Company.

Palmer, J.A. (2009). Nursing research: understanding the basics. *Plastic Surgical Nursing, 29*(2), 115-121.

Polit, D.F., & Hungler, B.P. (1995). *Nursing Research Principles and Methods*, (5th ed.). Philadelphia: JB Lippincott Company.

Roberts, P., & Priest, H. (2006). Reliability and validity in research. *Nursing Standard*, *20*(44), 41-45.

Robinson Kurpius, S.E., & Stafford, M.E. (2005). *Testing and Measurement, A User-Friendly Guide*. London: Sage.

Salmond, S. (2008). Evaluating the Reliability and Validity of Measurement Instruments. *Orthopaedic Nursing*, 27(1), 28-30.

Shrout, P. E., & Fleiss, J. L. (1979). Intra-class correlations: uses in assessing rater reliability. *Psychological Bulletin, 86* (2), 420-422.

Utwin, M.S. (1995). *How to Measure Survey Reliability and Validity*. Thousand Oaks: Sage Publications.

Yen, M.F., & Lo, L.H. (2002). Examining test-retest reliability: an intra-class correlation approach. *Nursing Research, 51*(1), 59-62.

In: Nursing Research: A Chinese Perspective
Editor: Zenobia C. Y. Chan

ISBN: 978-1-61209-833-3
©2011 Nova Science Publishers, Inc.

Chapter XVII

Measure with a Reliable Ruler: Choose a Reliability Test for Your Nursing Research

S. T. Wong and Zenobia C. Y. Chan

The Hong Kong Polytechnic University, China

Summary

Various research literature authors mention many reliability tests to be done before using an instrument in a research. However, most of them do not explain the situations and limitations in using them so that many new researchers are confused when trying to estimate the reliability of the instrument. In this article, a comprehensive review on literature about reliability of nursing research is done to explain the principles of using different reliability tests and the limitations of using these tests. Using a suitable reliability test for the instrument of a research can increase the efficiency to start carrying out a research.

In the research field, instruments help to record and collect data from the samples according to Boswell and Cannon (2007). Questionnaires, biophysical instruments and even people can be instruments for data collection in a research. Quantitative data isare numerical; therefore, the instruments for data collection in quantitative research are mainly questionnaires, rating scales, checklists, standardized tests and biophysical measures (Fain, 2009). For nursing research, questionnaires, scales and biophysical instruments may be mostly used.

Reliability of data collection instruments in research is also important. The reliability of a quantitative measure is a major criterion for assessing its quality (Polit & Hungler, 1997). For example, we use a thermometer to measure temperature of 2 glasses of water. Suppose they are at the same temperature; the same readings should be expected to be observed. However, if the readings are different, how can we trust the results obtained by this unreliable instrument? Applying to research, if the data collection instrument gives you different readings even when the actual results remain constant, people will not trust the research findings and the research becomes meaningless. Burns and Grove (2005) state that reliable instruments can enhance the power of a research by showing the actual relationships between the variables under study. With better reliability, the results of the research will be more accurate and trustworthy. Therefore, it is important to test the reliability of an instrument before using it in a study. However, most of authors (Dempsey & Dempsey, 2000; Fain, 2009; Lobiondo-wood & Haber, 2009; Nieswiadomy, 1998; Parahoo, 1997; Polit & Hungler, 1997; Seaman, 1987; Treece & Treece, 2001) treat reliability as less than a chapter or just a paragraph. New researchers generally do not get a clear picture on reliability like why to use that reliability test and what the differences are between the tests. It will take them a lot of time to read from different sources in order to find out if the instrument is reliable or not. This article is to save their time and cost to find out which instrument should be used andwhile which should not be used due to its unreliability.

When deciding what instruments are to be used, LoBiondo-Wood and Haber (2009) suggests that literature review be conducted as researchers can explore how other researchers measure the similar variables of interest and can see whether the existing instruments can be adapted in the current research. However, not every research is are suitable to use an existing instrument. New instruments and modified existing instruments are sometimes used. Should there be no suitable instruments existing, researchers may have to develop a new instrument on their own. Before applying an existing reliable instrument in the present research, reliability tests are a must. Burns and Grove (2005) mentioned that high reliability on an existing instrument does not guarantee its reliability will be good enough in another sample or with a different population. For example, researchers carry out a research on 'stress' by using the same questionnaire on adolescent and adults. Adults and adolescents are in different populations so reliability tests should be done to see if the questionnaire is reliable on both groups. Researchers may sometimes need to add or delete some items to or from the existing instruments. These actions may alter the reliability of the instruments according to Nieswiadomy (1998). Therefore, reliability testing is always needed to be conducted no matter when choosing an existing instrument or developing a new instrument. By conducting a pilot study for the present sample, according to Lobiondo-wood and Haber (1998), can determine if the instruments being used later are reliable or not. A Ppilot study helps researchers to test the applicability of the sample and also the instrument of the research in an efficient way without actually carrying out a research.

Stability, homogeneity and equivalence are the main concerns while testing reliability. Each of these elements has its own tests to measure itself. Choosing a reliability test suitable for a research can save time so that researchers can start collecting data as soon as possible rather than spending a large portion of their time on deciding which instrument to use.

Reliability testing focuses on three main aspects including stability, homogeneity and equivalence (Fain, 2009). In a nutshell, stability means the extent in which the same results arebe obtained on repeated applications of the instrument (Polit & Hungler, 1999); homogeneity describes the extent that items in the instrument measure different aspects of the same concept (Fink, 1995) ; equivalence refers to the extent that the same results arebe obtained when equivalent or parallel instruments are used (Lobiondo-wood & Haber, 1998). However, not all of these three aspects have to be used to assess an instrument because the aspect might not be important for the instrument, but at least one of the aspects has to be tested to show the instrument is reliable to be used in a research. The comparison of these three reliability tests will be shown in Table 1.

Table 1. Comparison of reliability tests

	Stability	Homogeneity	Equivalence
Descriptions	The extent that the same results arebe obtained on repeated applications of the instrument	The extent that items in the instrument measures different aspects of the same concept	The extent that the same results arebe obtained when equivalent or parallel instruments are used
Situations to be used	The instrument will be used more than once in a research	The instrument is intentionally examining one concept or construct at a time	More than one forms of instruments or more than one observer or rater are used in the research
Tests used	Test-retest reliability	Split-half technique	Inter-rater
		Cronbach's alpha	Alternate forms
		Kuder– Richardson formula 20 (KR-20)	

Stability Reliability (Test-Retest Reliability)

The use of Stability Reliability

Stability reliability, also called test-retest reliability, is used when measurement over time is the concern (LoBiondo-Wood & Haber, 2009), for example, researchers carry out a longitudinal study or want to test the change on a variable after an intervention. Thus, when an instrument is used to collect data more than once in a research, a stable instrument over time is important. Stability reliability is used to assess the stability of the instrument. According to Parahoo (1997), stability reliability is administering the same instrument, usually the questionnaire and scales, to the same individuals similar to the ones the researchers plans to study, on two occasions and comparing the responses. Suppose a researcher tests the stability of a self-administered questionnaire about stress faced by nurses. The questionnaire will be distributed and administered to a group of nurses and it is re-administered again to the same group of nurses after a period of time, for example, a month. By adding up the scores of each item in the instrument, the first and second total score can be calculated for each sample. If the difference between the two scores is very narrow or even none, the instrument can be said to pass the test-retest and, be stable and so reliable (Parahoo, 1997). The two scores are then correlated statistically to get a correlation coefficient (ranged from .00 to 1) called the coefficient of stability, usually a Pearson r (Dempsey & Dempsey, 2000). The higher the coefficient shows the more stable the measure (Bannigan & Watson, 2009). Generally speaking, the second scores should not be different from the first scores if there is nothing happened to change the attitudes of the individuals. If there is a change, the result of the stability test is untrustworthy. If nothing happened but the two scores are different, the instrument is not stable.

Limitation of Stability Reliability

The time interval between two administrations of the instrument can be a big question for researchers. It varies from a few days to several months or even longer. Should the interval be too short, the individuals may remember their responses on the first administration and give an over-estimation of reliability. Should it be too long, changes may occur withon the individual during the time interval between two administrations and give an under-estimation of reliability.

    a)   Overestimation of stability reliability

If the time between two administrations is short, individuals who takes the test may remember their responses at the first testing time. Mclaughlin and Marascuilo (1990) mention that the shorter the time interval between the first and second administration of the same instrument, the greater the probability that patients will recall their initial responses and give it again. This results in an artificially high coefficient of reliability no matter if the instrument is reliable or not.

    b)   Underestimation of stability reliability

As mentioned before, changes in attitude of the samples may occur between the two administrations. With the above example of nurses' stress, if there are some rules and regulations imposed to the nurses during the period, they will become more stressful at the second administration and their answers to the questionnaire will be different. Their answers change independently of the stability of the instrument over time. If the factor being measured does change, the test is not a measure of reliability. Therefore, the instrument may be reliable but the change decreases the stability of the questionnaire which is the under-estimation of the reliability.

Therefore, the time interval should be long enough to let individuals forget their responses in the first test but not long enough for the individuals to change. The interval is usually two to three weeks (Young, Taylor & Renpenning, 2001). Attitudes, mood, knowledge, physical condition, etc. are some common items of interest change over time (Polit & Hungler, 1997). They can change markedly during the period of time. Therefore, stability reliability may not be the appropriate type of reliability for these traits. Nevertheless, if some relatively enduring characteristics like self-esteem, personality and abilities are tested, the stability test result is more trustworthy.

Homogeneity Reliability
(Internal Consistency Reliability)

The use of Homogeneity Reliability

Homogeneity reliability, also called internal consistency reliability, is appropriate only when the instrument is intentionally examining one concept or construct at a time (Nieswiadomy, 1998). Therefore, if the instrument is examining more than one concept, this homogeneity cannot be the reliability test for the instrument. However, it is convenient for the researchers to use the homogeneity test to estimate the reliability of an instrument (Dempsey & Dempsey, 2000). It, unlike the test-retest reliability, requires only one administration to the individuals; besides, it, unlike the alternate-form test, requires only one form of the instrument. According to Bannigan and Watson (2009), procedures for measuring homogeneity include the 'split-half technique', 'Cronbach's alpha' (or 'coefficient alpha') and the 'Kuder– Richardson formula 20' (KR-20). As statistical tests can be used to test the homogeneity reliability, time can be saved.

Split-Half

The items in an instrument are divided into two equal halves by the question numbers: odd and even numbers or first part and second part or by random allocation. The sum of each halfve of each individual is calculated and then a correlation coefficient between the two sums is computed (LoBiondo-Wood & Haber, 2009). If the instrument is internally homogenous, the sum of the two halves should be approximately equal and the correlation coefficient should be high, tends to 1.00 (Seaman, 1987). This means that the items in the instrument are measuring the same attitude.

Limitations of Split-Half

If the instrument is split into halves in different approaches, comparing odd- and even or first and second halves, the correlation coefficient may be different. Boswell and Cannon (2007) suggest the items be matched between each half, based on the content and difficulty. However, it takes a lot of time to allocate the questions and difficulty may be different in the perspective of researchers and different samples. Burns and Grove (2005) suggest that researchers split the instrument in different possible ways and conduct the correlation tests for each split then average the coefficient to obtain one correlation coefficient. LoBiondo-Wood and Haber (2009) suggest an item-to-total correlation in which the relationship between each of the items and the total scale is measured. When item-to-total correlations are calculated, a correlation for each item is generated. Items that do not achieve a high correlation may be deleted from the instrument. However, both of the above suggestions are time consuming. Dempsey and Dempsey (2000) suggest usinge Cronbach's alpha (coefficient alpha) which allows the researcher to compare the results of each item on an instrument with every other item and average the results to achieve a correlation coefficient. This correlation coefficient is the average of all of the possible split-half reliabilities of an instrument when the responses to the questions on the instrument can be scored as having several possible responses. Among these suggestions, using Cronbach's alpha seems to be the best. It saves researchers time to divide the items in the instrument and at the same time, it calculates and draws a mean for the coefficients.

For items that are responded to in a Likert scale or dichotomous response, other methods are used. These methods are also used to examine the extent to which all of the items in the instrument measure the same concept, like the test-retest.

Cronbach's Alpha

Cronbach's alpha (coefficient alpha) not only can be used to correlate the split-half test but can also be used with instruments composed of items that can be scored with 3 or more possible values. For example, with the Likertk scale used commonly in measuring psychosocial variables, the question is on a scale of different degrees of intensity between two extremes, like 'strongly agree' to 'agree' to 'no comment' to 'disagree' to 'strongly disagree'; the points between the two extremes may range from 1 to 5 or 1 to 7 (LoBiondo-Wood & Haber, 2009). To test the reliability of the scales, researchers administer an instrument to a group of individuals then all responses are scored, Cronbach' alpha is applied to compare each item in the scale with the others (Fain, 2009).

Kr-20

Another method to estimate homogeneity reliability is the KR-20. According to Dempsey and Dempsey (2000), KR-20 is a special case of Cronbach's alpha and is used for instruments having dichotomous response format that is the 'true or false' and 'yes or no' responses. As with test-retest reliability coefficients, indexes of these two tests range in value between 0.00 and 1.00. The higher the reliability coefficient means the more internally consistent the measure is.

Limitations of Homogeneity Reliability

Homogeneity reliability tests are applicable primarily with paper and pencil tests; also, it can also only be used to test the reliability of an instrument which for measuring but not describing or exploring a phenomenon (Parahoo, 1997). It is obvious only that instruments with ordinal and interval measurements can use homogeneity reliability but it is not necessary paper and pencil tests; sometimes, observers are used as an instrument to observe the samples and give scores. Bannigan and Watson (2009) mention that the procedures for internal consistency do not consider fluctuations over time. The fluctuations over time should be tested by the stability reliability rather than homogeneity reliability.

Equivalence Reliability

The Use of Equivalence Reliability

Equivalence reliability can be used as a test for reliability when more than one forms of instrument or more than one observer or rater are used in the research. According to Burns and Grove (2005), equivalence reliability has two types: alternate forms reliability and inter-rater reliability. The former one is done by administering and comparing two parallel forms of the same instrument or two instruments to the same sample while the latter one is by administering and comparing the same form by different raters or observers (Bannigan & Watson, 2009). Therefore, equivalence reliability is to test the consistency of different instruments to determine whether the instruments provide the same result when collecting the same data.

Interr-Rater Reliability

Inter-rater reliability is often used in structured observational instruments because direct observation can reduce its reliability due to observer error and the reliability test is to assess the degree of error (Polit & Hubler, 1997). When two or more researchers participate as observers or raters (data collectors) observing or rating the situation and recording the observations, using the same record format independently in a research, inter-rater reliability has to be done (Parahoo, 1997). This is to quantify the degree of consistency among raters and observers. The resulting data can then be used to calculate to demonstrate the strength of the relation between the ratings of the two observers. According to Fain (2009), one popular statistical procedure that quantifies the degree of consistency among raters is called Cohen's kappa which is used in nominal data (discreet categories). If all raters agree that a particular item belongs in a given category and there is total agreement for all items being evaluated, then Cohen's Kkappa assumes the value of 1.0. The values range from .00 to 1.00, higher value indicates a greater degree of equivalence.

Alternate Forms Reliability

According to Dempsey and Dempsey (2000), at least 2 different forms of the instrument are constructed that each form has the same number of total test items, is designed to measure the same variable or variables, and has the same level of difficulty, although the actual items on the instruments are not the same. Nieswiadomy (1998) reminds that one form of the test is administered to a group of people and the other form is administered either at the same time or shortly thereafter to these same people. A correlation coefficient (coefficient of equivalence) is obtained between the two forms. The higher the coefficient, tending to 1, means the higher equivalence reliability. The two forms can be altered by changing the order of categories or substituting the wordings used in one form by the same meaning equivalent terms to generate a new form.

Limitation of Equivalence Reliability

For the inter-rater reliability, when raters know they are being watched, their accuracy and consistency are considerably better than when they believe they are not being watched (Lobiondo-wood & Haber, 1998). Thus, the inter-rater reliability will be overestimated. However, if the reliability test is done secretly, the true value of interr-rater reliability can be assessed. For the alternate forms of reliability, it is difficult to construct two forms of instruments that are exactly equivalent and to administer two different instruments to the same individuals within a relatively short period of time (Dempsey & Dempsey, 2000). It will cost a lot of energy and time to generate a new equivalent form.

Conclusion

Reliability values must be included in published reports of the study according to Burns and Grove (2005). There must be at least one reliability test applicable for the instrument. Many reliability tests are mentioned above but researchers may not have enough time to conduct all of the tests. Here are some guidelines for you to follow. If there is only one form of research instrument or no more than one observer or rater in the research, equivalence reliability can be ignored. If the items in the instrument are not supposed to measure the same trait, for example, it measures both the behavior and mood of the samples, homogeneity reliability can be ignored. The most applicable one may be the stability reliability but it may not be meaningful if the instrument is administered only once during the research. Whatever the reliability test is used, when the reliability coefficient is below 0.80, researchers may need to amend the items in the existing instrument; some may even have to find or develop another instrument for the research. Without a reliable instrument, a research cannot be started to carry out. If the research is carried out with an unstable instrument, the research will be untrustworthy and the time and cost spent on the research is a kind of wasted. Therefore, determining the reliability of an instrument is an important step for starting a research.

Author's Background

Wong Sin Tung, a year two student who is studying Master of Nursing in Hong Kong Polytechnic University and the Hong Kong Sanatorium Hospital and graduated from Bachelor of Arts in Hong Kong Shue Yan University. (Email: sin74tung@gmail.com)

References

Bannigan, K. & Watson, R. (2009). Reliability and validity in a nutshell. *Journal of Clinical Nursing, 18,* 3237-3243.

Boswell, C. & Cannon, S. (2007). *Introduction to nursing research: Incorporating evidence-based practice.* Sudbury: Jones and Bartlett Publishers.

Boswell-Ruys, C. L., Sturnieks, D. L., Harvey, L. A., Sherrington, C., Middleton, J. W. & Lord, S. R. (2009). Validity and reliability of assessment tools for measuring unsupported sitting in people with a spinal cord injury. *Archives of Physical Medicine & Rehabilitation, 90,* 1571-1577.

Burns, N. & Grove, S. K. (2005). *The practice of nursing research: Conduct, critique, and utilization.* St. Louis: Elsevier/Saunders.

Dempsey, P. A. & Dempsey, A. D. (2000). *Using nursing research: Process, critical evaluation, and utilization.* Philadelphia: Lippincott.

De Vera, M. A., Ratzlaff, C., Doerfling, P. & Kopec, J. (2010). Reliability and validity of an internet-based questionnaire measuring lifetime physical activity. *American Journal of Epidemiology, 172* (10), 1190-1198.

Fain, J. A. & (2009). *Reading, understanding, and applying nursing research.* Philadelphia: F.A. Davis Co.

Fink, A. (1995). *The Survey kit.* Thousand Oaks: Sage Publications.

Kimberlin, C. L. & Winterstein, A. G. (2008). Validity and reliability of measurement instruments used in research. *American Journal of Health-system Pharmacy, 65,* 2276-2284.

Kring, D. L. (2007). Reliability and validity of the Braden Scale for predicting pressure ulcer.*Journal of Wound, Ostomy & Continence Nursing, 34*(4), 399-406.

Lobiondo-wood, G. & Haber, J. (1998). *Nursing research: Methods, critical appraisal, and utilization.* St. Louis: Mosby.

Lobiondo-wood, G. & Haber, J. (2009). *Nursing research in Canada: Methods and critical appraisal for evidence-based practice.* Toronto: Mosby Elsevier.

Mclaughlin, F. E. & Marascuilo, L. A. (1990). *Advanced nursing and health care research: Quantification approaches,* Philadelphia: Saunders.

Nieswiadomy, R. M. (1998). *Foundations of nursing research.* Stamford: Appleton & Lange.

Parahoo, K. (1997). *Nursing research: principles, process and issues.* Basingstoke: Macmillan.

Paternostro-Sluga, T.,Grim-Stieger, M., Posch, M., Schuhfried, O., Vacariu, G., Mittermaier, C., Bittner, C. & Fialka-Moser, V. (2008). Reliability and validity of the Medical Research Council (MRC) scale and a modified scale for testing muscle strength in patients with radial palsy. *Journal of Rehabilitation Medicine, 40*(8), 665-671.

Polit, D. F. & Hungler, B. P. (1997). *Essentials of nursing research: Methods, appraisals, and utilization.* Philadelphia: Lippincott-Raven.

Polit, D. F. & Hungler, B. P. (1999). *Nursing Research Principles and Methods.* Philadelphia: JB Lippincott Company.

Seaman, C. H. C. (1987). *Research methods: Principles, practice, and theory for nursing,* Norwalk: Appleton & Lange.

Treece, E. W. & Treece, J. W. (2001). *Elements of research in nursing.* St. Louis: Mosby.

Wilson, H. S. (1989). *Research in nursing.* Redwood City: Addison-Wesley.

Yawn, B. P. & Wollan, P. (2005). Interrater reliability: completing the methods description in medical records review studies. *American Journal of Epidemiol, 161,* 974-977.

Young, A., Taylor, S. G. & Mclaughlin-renpenning, K. (2001). *Connections: Nursing research, theory, and practice.* St. Louis: Mosby.

Zenk, S. N., Schulz, A. J., Mentz, G., House, J. S., Gravlee, C. C., Miranda, P. Y., Miller, P. & Kannan, S. (2007). Inter-rater and test-retest reliability*Health & Place, 13*(2), 452-465.

In: Nursing Research: A Chinese Perspective
Editor: Zenobia C. Y. Chan

ISBN: 978-1-61209-833-3
©2011 Nova Science Publishers, Inc.

Chapter XVIII

Make Friends with Qualitative Research

I. M. Lam and Zenobia C. Y. Chan
The Hong Kong Polytechnic University, China

Summary

Qualitative research allows finding out the detailed information from the human society. It includes various approaches such as phenomenology, ethnography, case study and grounded theory. Each of them has their own characteristics to contribute to different research problems and objectives. Familiarizing with different types of research and choosing the most appropriate one for the research is important. This essay introduces the qualitative research and phenomenology, ethnography, case study and grounded theory based on the literature review. In addition, I will also express my preference of one research method - ethnography. This essay aims at providing a brief introduction about the qualitative research for who may be the first time to encountering qualitative research for the first time. I hope qualitative research will become your friend and you would like to know it more.

Introduction

Background

Research is applied in various fields such as biology, medicine, nursing and psychology with different purposes. It is generally is used for describing, explaining and predicting about a thing, an event or a phenomenon and hence, our scopes and lives are broadened (Marczyk, DeMatteo & Festinger, 2005). Based on what the researchers need, conducting a research can be achieved by using qualitative or quantitative research. Each of them can affect how the research is done. For example, the data collection tools and the data analysis may become different. In this essay, qualitative research will be introduced.

Objective

This essay does not aim at showing how to write a qualitative research. Instead, it is just going to let the novices at researcher obtain the basic knowledge and information about the qualitative research and understand the purposes of using qualitative research. This essay also lets the novices distinguish between different qualitative research methods and understand the advantages and limitations of using qualitative research. Therefore, the novices can be equipped well for stepping into the further learning of qualitative research.

Qualitative research is a research to be encountered all the time. In order to conduct a qualitative research with high quality, choosing the appropriate research method is essential.

In this essay, the literature review about the use and the reasons of using qualitative research will be provided. Then, four major qualitative research methods (phenomenology, ethnography, case study and grounded theory) are introduced as well. Then, the advantages and limitations will be discussed and finally, I will show which one of the four qualitative research methods is my preference.

Make Friends with Qualitative Research

How many friends do you have? How do you get familiar with them? Do you remember the first time you met them and how is it? For the first time of meeting with your friends, the first impression that comes to you may be the outlook appearance. In this essay, a friend called qualitative research will be introduced in the way like how what you observe your friends for the first time.

What is Qualitative Research?

Research is done through making sense of the evidence to create new knowledge and this evidence is found from the scientific research (Gillham, 2000). When the journey of conducting research is initiated, two basic forms of research may be heard all the time. They are quantitative and qualitative research. Quantitative research is an approach of collecting numerical data to find out the answer for the research question through statistical analysis (Christensen, Johnson, & Turner, 2011; Marczyk, DeMatteo, & Festinger, 2005). On the other hand, the qualitative research method can give us a detailed description and analysis of human experience and the explanation of the phenomena in the research (Marvasti, 2004; Hansen, 2006). In other words, quantitative research focuses on statistical numbers while qualitative research focuses more on the descriptive words (number v.s. word). Both of them are used in different situations based what the research questions are.

Hansen (2006) stated that all qualitative researches belonged to social research but might not be vice versa. Social research means the research related to the human behavior and the social life (Berg, 2004). In addition, Stake (2010) used few characteristics to describe the qualitative research, which were interpretive, experiential, situational and personalistic. As a result, the detailed and descriptive analysis is usually is found and all the findings and resultse should be socially related to the human life experience and the society in qualitative research.

Once either the qualitative or the quantitative research is selected, the goal of research will be achieved through the different processes such as a data collection tool, sample size, data analysis. It is very important to choose the appropriate approach to conduct the research. But why do we choose qualitative research? The most important consideration is whether it is suitable for responding the research problem (Hansen, 2006). It may be also due to the personal passion, desire for in-depth information, research problem limitation (answer must be found through qualitative research methods) and even other constrictions such as funding (Warren & Karner, 2010). Other factors for choosing a particular research approach may be affected by the researcher's point of view to the world, personality, the researcher's disciplinary background and the institution the research is working for and the preference of the research's audience (Blaikie, 1993). Furthermore, before choosing qualitative research, based on Punch (1998) mentioned, we could think whether this method is suitable to answer the research questions; whether the detail information is needed; how the researches with related topics were done by others; whether enough resources and access is obtained for conducting the research; which method make us learn more. In addition, what kind of the data is required to respond to the research problem, descriptive information or numerical data? Considering the above factors and questions may help us to decide whether qualitative research method should be chosen for the research.

Table 1. Summary table of phenomenology, ethnography, case study and grounded theory

	Phenomenology	Ethnography	Case Study	Grounded Theory
Function	Understanding the human experience	Description of a group, culture or community	Intensive study of case	Developing a theory by using qualitative data inductively
Data Collection	In-depth interview Open-ended questionnaire	In-depth interview Participant observation (overt & covert)	Interview Questionnaire Archival records	Interview observation
Features	Entering participants' inner world Participants' perspective Bracket pre-conception of researcher's mind Descriptive Experience Unique live experience	Emic and etic perspective Culture Contact with participants Going native Researchers acting like a participant	In-depth study Exploration of participants- issues relationship "how" or "why" questions Intrinsic, instrumental and collective case	Concurrent process of data collection & analysis Modifying theory allowed in future Theory application Theory development

Four Major Qualitative Research Methods

Christensen, Johnson, and Turner (2011) mentioned that qualitative research was a broad form of research and it included at least four major methods to conduct a qualitative research, including phenomenology, ethnography, case study and grounded theory. The features between these four qualitative research methods is shown in Table 1.

- Phenomenology

Phenomenology is a discovery method to understand the human experience through the description of the phenomenon (Parse, 2001). Lived experience is an important element in phenomenology (Rossman & Rallis, 2003). The researcher steps into the life world of the participants in order to obtain the valuable information and the tools of data collection are usually are in-depth interviews and open-ended questionnaires (Christensen, Johnson, & Turner, 2011). The information given by the participants are from their point of view and the researchers need to bracket their pre-conceptions to understand the participants' experience (Gray, 2009). It means the researchers should obtain the data with an objective attitude and without being contaminated by their subjective view. In phenomenology, the experience is described rather than being defined or explained (Hek & Moule, 2006). Each of the individuals' experience is unique although the participants are undergoing the same situation or phenomenon. This kind of experience is expected to come from the participants' real life and may not be obtained in detail through the quantitative research. merely.

- Ethnography

Ethnography focuses on the description of a group, culture or community and the data collection methods include interviews, participant observations and even the documents such as diaries (Holloway & Wheeler, 2010). Participant observation includes overt or covert participant observation: overt participant observation means the participants know they are being observed while covert participant observation means they do not know about it (Gray, 2009). Since culture is so important in ethnography, familiarizing the participants' culture or the events is are essential to conduct a comprehensive and more accurate research. There are two different views to describe the participants' culture. They are insider's perspective (emic perspective) and objective outsider's perspective (etic perspective) and both of them should be balanced in conducting the research (Christensen, Johnson, & Turner, 2011). Insider's perspective can be obtained by the researcher's understanding of the participants' life through actually experiencing as a participant (going native) (Hek & Moule, 2006). On the other hand, outsider's perspective can be gained from social science theory and the researcher's experience (Rossman & Rallis, 2003).

- Case Study

Case study centers on the intensive study of the varied cases such as the person or the event (Glesne, 2011). It is descriptive, holistic, heuristic and inductive (Rossman & Rallis, 2003). Case study can be used for exploring the ambiguous relationship between the participants and issues (Gray, 2009). It is good for being used when the "how" or "why" questions are asked (Yin, 2003). Case studies can be obtained from in-depth interviews, questionnaires or archival records (Christensen, Johnson, & Turner, 2011). Stake (1995) mentioned three types of case study which were called intrinsic, instrumental and collective study: intrinsic case study is not the case studied with interest for the purpose of learning the general problem, but it is for the need to learn the particular case and this is called intrinsic interest; instrumental case study is to give insight into an issue and facilitate our understanding of something else; collective case study is like instrumental case study but multiple cases were selected for understanding the problem. So, case study is like a way to widen our scope to the issue. It sometimes may give us the indication or the clue to find out the answer for the issue.

- **Grounded Theory**

Grounded theory is a method to generate and develop a theory by using qualitative data inductively (from specific moving to general) (Charmaz, 2001). Other than generating a new theory, existing theories can also be modified (Holloway & Wheeler, 2010). Theory should be discovered in the working field or empirical data rather than applied to the participants (Flick, 2009). Christensen, Johnson, and Turner, (2011) mentioned that the common method of data collection was the interview, and followed by observation and the researcher was required to have a good perception of which data is important and decide the need for obtaining more additional data for the research. Hence, the data may need to be integrated and verified afor few times so as to know whether the existing data is enough, appropriate and relevant. Besides, in grounded theory research, data collection and data analysis are interrelated and should be proceeded concurrently because it facilitates the subsequent data collection (Bryant & Charmaz, 2007; Corbin & Stauss, 1990). Therefore, based on the data analysis, some adjustment may need to be done for the next data collection so as to obtain the more accurate and useful data.

According to Glaser and Strauss (1967), there are four interrelated properties for using grounded theory: the theory should be fit for use, understandable by laymen, generally applicable to diverse situations and partial control of the situations. As a result, if the theory is found that does not fit in with these four properties during the conducting of the research, the reason should be investigated and it should be considered whether the correction or extra data isare needed for the research.

Discussions

Other than the point of the above four methods that can be used in qualitative research, some other parts of them are quite similar. For example, data collection methods such as interviews areis used. The researcher themself can be the instrument for collecting the data and has direct contact with the participants in those four methods. Besides, detailed data can be obtained and thatose data may come from the subjective view of the participants. Furthermore, four methods can also be applied in nursing or health-care research. The examples such as the researches were done by Spichiger (2010), Cricco-Lizza (2009), Ma and Waddington (1998) and Lalor, Begley and Devane (2006). On the other hand, the focus of four methods is different. For example, phenomenology, ethnology, case study and grounded theory center on human experience, culture, intensive study one or more cases and developing theory, respectively.

Qualitative research method is a good approach when someone's experience is described. Data can be obtained from the participants by listening, even experiencing or feeling what they had experienced. As comparing with the quantitative research, the in-depth or elaborated sharing from the participants may not be gained in quantitative research.

However, everything has its own advantages and limitations. It is the same as qualitative research. For the advantages, the in-depth data can be obtained through different data collection methods and the abundant descriptions may be generated by the reflection of participant's reality (Gills & Jackson, 2002). Even the research can obtain much further information from the participants based on their responses. On the other hand, as compared with other research methods, qualitative research is weaker in objectivity and generabiliy because the sample size is too small and data collected isare too familiarized by the researcher and this makes the researcher quite subjective to conduct the research, such as in the aspect of sample selected and data analysis (Gills & Jackson, 2002). Besides, some processes in research such as data collection and data transcription are quite time-consuming.

If you let me choose my favorite qualitative research method, I will choose ethnography. It is because ethnographic research can allow having a close interaction with the participants through real experience in their society. Ethnographic research can not only obtain the information from listening to the participants' experience, but also let me personally experience what those participants experience and observe how they act in their daily lives. This is an observation overin a long period of time rather than a short time. It provides an opportunity to experience the change and the development between people to people within a human society. It also gives more time for establishing the relationship with the participants and I think the relationship is helpful in obtaining more in-depth information from the participants. Furthermore, ethnography allows me to think about what I gain and why there is any similar or different feelings produced from the experience of acting as the participant. Hence, it can help me to familiarize more about the participants' context which may contribute to the reflection of their experience. Besides, I can also learn the culture and the behavior personally from the participants simultaneously rather than merely understand it from the books and words, so that it can impress and broaden my vision. In addition, I think by going native, this behavior can enhance the empathy, which is also an important attitude in nursing. This will foster my quality of care to the patients based on their need and view if using ethnography in health care.

Conclusion

The most important thing about whether qualitative research should be used in the research depends on whether it can correspond and suit to the research problem. Phenomenology, ethnography, case study and grounded theory are the qualitative research methods. Each of them serves to different purposes in the research. Phenomenology is for finding the significance in the people under the same phenomenon; ethnography is for research the finding from the culture in the human society; case study is for having a more in-depth understanding of the cases; grounded theory is for developing the theory to explain the phenomena. In addition, conducting qualitative research can obtain the in-depth and broader information from the participants but it is quite time-consuming and some people may think the particular selected small sample size by the researcher is a problem regarding to the objectivity and generability. However, conducting research is not just for answering the research question, but what is learnedt is also important. This essay only provides a very brief introduction to qualitative research. If you want to know more about this friend, please search and learn from more related literatures and even try to start your journey in qualitative research at the same time.

Author's Background

Lam Io Man, Elmon, a year two student who is studying the second degree in Master of Nursing in the Hong Kong Polytechnic University and, a graduate student from Institute for Tourism Studies in Macau for the first degree in Bachelor of Science in Hotel Management. (Email: elmon_im@yahoo.com.hk)

References

Berg, B. L. (2004). *Qualitative research methods for the social sciences* (5th ed.). Boston, MA: Pearson/Allyn and Bacon.

Blaikie, N. W. H. (1993). *Approaches to social enquiry*. Cambridge: Polity Press.

Bryant, A., & Charmaz, K. (2007). Introduction grounded theory research: methods and practices. In A. Bryant & K. Charmaz (Eds.), *The Sage handbook of grounded theory* (pp. 1-28). London: SAGE.

Cricco-Lizza, R. (2009). Formative infant feeding experiences and education of NICU nurses. *American Journal of Maternal Child Nursing. 34*(4), 236-242.

Charmaz, K. (2001). Grounded theory analysis. *In J. F. Gubrium & J. A. Holstein (Eds.), Handbook of interviewing*, pp. 675-694. Thousand Oaks, CA: SAGE.

Christensen, L. B., Johnson, R. B., & Turner, L. A. (2011). *Research methods, design, and analysis* (11th ed.). Boston, MA: Allyn & Bacon/Pearson.

Corbin, J., & Strauss, A. (1990). Grounded theory research: procedures, canons, and evaluative criteria. *Qualitative Sociology, 13*(1), 153-169.

Flick, U. (2009). *An introduction to qualitative research* (4th ed.). London: SAGE Publication.

Gillham, B (2000). *Case study research methods*. London: Continuum.

Gillis, A., & Jackson, W. (2002). *Research for nurses: methods and interpretation*. Philadelphia, Pa.: F.A. Davis Co.

Glaser, B. G., & Strauss, A. L. (1967). *The discovery of grounded theory: strategies for qualitative research*. New York: Aldine Pubulishing Company.

Glesne, C. (2011). *Becoming qualitative researchers: an introduction* (4th ed.). Boston: Pearson.

Gray, D. E. (2009). *Doing research in the real world* (2nd ed.). London: SAGE Publications.

Hansen, E. C. (2006). *Successful qualitative health research: a practical introduction*. Maidenhead, England: Open University Press.

Hek, G., & Moule, P. (2006). *Making Sense of Research: An introduction for health and social care practitioners* (3rd ed.). London: SAGE Publications Ltd.

Holloway, I., & Wheeler, S. (2010). *Qualitative research in nursing and healthcare* (3rd ed.). Ames, Iowa: Wiley-Blackwell.

Lalor, J. G., Begley, C. M., & Devane, D. (2006). Exploring painful experiences: impact of emotional narratives on members of a qualitative research team. *Journal of Advanced Nursing, 56*(6), 607-616.

Ma, S. G., & Waddington, K. (1998). Role transition from staff nurse to clinical nurse specialist: a case study. *Journal of Clinical Nursing, 7,* 283-290.

Marczyk, G., DeMatteo, D., & Festinger, D. (2005). *Essentials of research design and methodology*. Hoboken, NJ: John Wiley & Sons.

Marvasti, A. B. (2004). *Qualitative research in sociology: an introduction*. London: SAGE Publications.

Parse, R. R. (2001). *Qualitative inquiry: the path of sciencing*. Boston: Jones and Bartlett Publisher.

Punch, K. F. (1998). *Introduction to social research: quantitative and qualitative Aapproaches*. London: Sage Publications.

Rossman, G. B., & Rallis, S. F. (2003). *Learning in the field: an introduction to qualitative research* (2nd ed.). Thousand Oaks, Calif.: SAGE Publications.

Spichiger, E. (2010). Patients' and families' experience of their relationship with professional healthcare providers in hospital end-of-life care: an interpretive phenomenological study. *Journal of Hospice and Palliative Nursing, 12*(3), 194-202.

Stake, R. E. (1995). *The art of case study research*. Thousand Oaks, Calif.: Sage Publications.

Stake, R. E. (2010). *Qualitative research: studying how things work*. New York: Guilford Press.

Warren, C. A. B., & Karner, T. X. (2010). *Discovering qualitative methods: field research, interviews, and analysis* (2nd ed.). New York: Oxford University Press.

Yin, R. K. (2003). *Case study research: design and methods* (3rd ed.). Thousand Oaks: SAGE Publications.

In: Nursing Research: A Chinese Perspective
Editor: Zenobia C. Y. Chan

ISBN: 978-1-61209-833-3
©2011 Nova Science Publishers, Inc.

Chapter XIX

Smart Ways to Recruit Informants for Qualitative Research

Karen T. Y. Chung and Zenobia C. Y. Chan
The Hong Kong Polytechnic University, China

Summary

Qualitative interviewing is a way of finding out what others feel and think about their worlds. We need to get in- depth information from the interviewees for analysis in qualitative research. A improper informant would speaks superficially or exaggerates the real experience for the sake of holding the researcher's attention and they may be unwilling to trust the interviewer and reveal his or her true feelings. Therefore, it is important to know how to choose the right people to interview who can provide credible information. Clear principles are important to guide us to choose proper informants. Purposive sampling and Ttheoretical sampling are often used in qualitative research. They have different criteria. Purposive sampling generally selects informants within extreme situations as for certain characteristics or informants with a wide range of situations in order to maximize variation (Gobo, 2004), while theoretical sampling selects groups or categories to study on the basis of their relevance to research questions and theoretical position, and most importantly, the explanation or account which we are developing (Mason, 1996). Regardless of the type of sample employed, informants must be selected or carefully chosen according to specific qualities (Agar, 1980; Hammersley & Atkinson, 1983; Morse, 1991)

Introduction

In qualitative interviewing, researchers need to request the interviewees to explore the questions in- depth. The researchers need to encourage the interviewees to reflect, in detail, on events they have experienced (Rubin & Rubin, 1995). It is shown that we need to get in-depth information from the interviewees for analysis in qualitative research. So how do we choose the right people to interview who can provide credible information?

Sampling is an unavoidable consideration because it is everyday life activity deeply rooted in thought, language and practice. After having specified a population, the researcher decides if he or she will collect information on all of its individuals or on a sub-set of cases (Gobo, 2004). In qualitative approaches, researchers demand different sampling techniques than the randomly selected and probabilistic sampling which quantitative researchers often use. The sampling strategies adopted can make a difference to the whole study (Holloway & Wheeler, 1996). Moreover, Morse (1991) also points out that the selection of a sample has a profound effect on the ultimate quality of the research. Therefore, it is important to think out exactly what our sampling strategy will be in order to choose proper informants. The following parts of the essay show you the details about the smart ways of sampling to help you recruit the right informants for conducting qualitative research with good quality. They are a) Principles of recruiting informants; b) Different criteria for choosing proper informants in different qualitative research methods; d) Qualities of good informants; e) Discussion.

The Study

1) Principles of Recruiting Informants

When doing qualitative research, we should be careful to recruit suitable informants in order to get good quality research. Clear principles are important to guide us to choose proper informants. Here are some relevant principles being listed.

According to Rubin & Rubin (1995), all of the people that you interview should satisfy three requirements generally. They should be knowledgeable about the cultural arena or the situation or experience being studied; they should be willing to talk; when people in the arena have different perspectives, the interviewees should represent the range of points of view.

In your early interviews, you can start with people whose job it is to monitor what goes on in that arena in order to sketch the overall situation. Then you can choose a number of people who represent specific factions or points of view. As you continue the research, you want to find other interviewees who can provide insights on more specific themes that emerge from the interviews. When interviewing people mentioned by previous interviewees, you make a start on interviewing along a social network. Networked introductions allow a study to begin, but the choices of the first person to interview may color the responses of later interviewees (Rubin & Rubin, 1995). It shows that the researchers may get one side of an argument only. It seems not sufficient to support the study.

We must go for balance in our choice of interviewees to represent all of the divisions within the area of study. By doing so, we can first test to see if similar themes and concepts hold elsewhere by interviewing people in arenas very much like those we have just examined. With a tougher test for generalization, dissimilarity sampling, we interview people with background characteristics different from those of our original interviewees, or we interview people in varying settings or who work in places other than the one you researched. When adding interviewees with diverse backgrounds, or in different situations, behave the same way or express the same values as our original interviewees, we gain confidence that what we have learned holds more broadly. Here is an example. "A nurse has decided that he wants to study patients' adherence to medical and nursing advice. His initial sample is patients from a surgical ward. He is interested in whether similar data could be collected from patients in a medical ward and therefore researches people in this setting." (Holloway & Wheeler, 1996). We can find that the nurse chose the relevant informants who were in the situation being studied and then he recruited some informants from another setting in order to test whether the people from the different setting behave the same way as his original interviewees and help him gain confidence that what he hasve learned holds more broadly.

Furthermore, in qualitative research, we need to know that the selection of an adequate and appropriate sample is also critical. Appropriateness means that the method of sampling fits the aim of the study and helps the understanding of the research problem. And when a sampling strategy is adequate, it generates adequate and relevant information and sufficient quality data (Holloway & Wheeler, 1996). It is clear to tell us that we have to choose proper informants and keep adding adequate informants who may come from different backgrounds in order to collect relevant data for supporting your study.

If we don't know clear guidelines on principles for the selection of a suitable sample, that may result in much confusion in the data collection process.

2) Different Criteria for Choosing Proper Informants in Different Qualitative Research Methods

Kuzel (1992) suggests five important characteristics of sampling in qualitative research: 1. Flexible sampling which develops during the study; 2. Sequential selection of sampling units; 3. Sampling guided by theoretical development which becomes progressively more focused; 4. Continuing sampling until no new relevant data arises; 5. Searching for negative or deviant cases. The selection of participants must be criterion-based, that is, certain criteria are applied, and the sample is chosen accordingly (Holloway & Wheeler, 1996). The criteria for selecting therefore, must be clearly identified.

Qualitative researchers are often interested in selecting purposive or judgment samples. The type of purposive sample chosen is based on the particular research question as well as consideration of the resources available to the research (Biber & Leavy, 2006). For example, "The purpose was to choose women that were as different as possible regarding social background, education, marital status and profession. Six were from the patient list of a physician, also one of the authors of this study and three participants who were not patients. Three of the nine participants were blue collar workers, two were well-paid administrators, two had sickness pensions and two were retired." The participants were purposefully chosen in accordance with the developing design [9]. (Lundqvist, Öhman & Weinehall, 2007)

Purposive sampling consists of detecting cases within extreme situations as for certain characteristics or cases with a wide range of situations in order to maximize variation, that is, to have all of the possible situations.(Gobo, 2004)(Qualitative Research Practice) Initially, the researcher may choose to interview informants with a broad, general knowledge of the topic or those who have undergone the experience and whose experience is considered typical. As the study progresses, the description is expanded with more specific information, and participants with that particular knowledge are deliberately sought. Finally, informants with atypical experiences are sought so that the entire range of experiences and the breadth of the concept or phenomena may be understood. (Morse, 1991)

The sample is selected according to the informants' knowledge of the research topic. It is essential for the researcher to discover who will be the most appropriate informant before beginning interviews. "A nurse researcher has been practicing in women's health for 12 years and wants to learn about the lived experiences of women needing hysterectomies. Experientially, this researcher has noticed an emotional difference in women with infertility who need hysterectomies versus fertile women who need hysterectomies. By narrowing the interest to women with infertility, the sample also narrows. If the researcher was interested in all women who need hysterectomies, the sample would include women from many ethnic groups, economic backgrounds, and age groups (e.g. adolescents, older adults). To adequately sample to understand the experiences of all patients needing hysterectomies, the researcher would need representative women from different ethnic groups, socioeconomic classes, and age groups." (Byme, 2001). We can find that the nurse researcher initially choose to interview informants with a broad, general knowledge of this topic. In order to adequately understand the experiences of all patients needing hysterectomies, the researcher selected the representative women from different ethnic groups, socioeconomic classes, and age groups. As the study progresses, the description is expanded with more specific information, and so participants who are women with infertility are deliberately sought.

Purposive sampling demands that we think critically about the parameters of the population we are studying and choose our sample case carefully on this basis. As Denzin and Lincoln (2000) said that many qualitative researchers employ purposive, and not random, sampling methods. They seek out groups, settings and individuals wheree…the processes being studied are mostly likely to occur.

Nurse ethnographers generally use purposive sampling which is criterion-based and non-probabilistic (Goetz & LeCompte, 1984). Ethnography involves describing and learning from a culture (Spradley, 1979). The sample is taken from a particular cultural or subcultural group. Ethnographers have to search for individuals within a culture who can give them specific detailed information about the culture. Ethnographers adopt certain criteria to choose a specific group and setting to be studied, be it a ward, a group of specialist nurses or patients with a specific condition (Hammersley & Atkinson, 1983). The criteria for sampling must be explicit and systematic, so proper informants can be selected.

Here is an example:. An in-depth qualitative research study was necessary to evaluate the opinions of the area's Latino population as well as the practices of healthcare providers in Washington County, Tennessee that provides care for the majority Caucasian population as well as Latino residents. The focus of this study was Latino patients that receive end of life care. For the research design, Eethnography was selected for this study. The constructs of the culture of Latino patients is studied to first determine what important rituals, traditions and beliefs surround the patient and families dealing with end of life issues. These constructs include issues such as treatment, pain control and religious rites. The researcher or their representative served as this ethnography's data collection instrument. For the Pparticipants., the study's sample represents a purposeful sampling of Latino patients receiving end-of-life care for various terminal illnesses. The researchers selected twenty two patients (fourteen male and eight female) from a Blood and Hematology Center; eleven patients (seven male and four female) from a university- based Cancer Center and five patients from Washington County, Tennessee that were enrolled in outpatient care with physicians (RByington, Grabner & Keene,2009). Using a purposeful sample which is a type of sampling in which the units to be observed are selected on the basis of the researcher's judgment will be the most useful or representative.

One of the main features of ethnography: work with key informants. Researchers should choose key informants carefully to make sure that they are suitable and representative of the group under study. Leininger (1985) said that a small sample of key informants can be more useful to the researcher than a large sample of general participants without specific knowledge of a topic. Key actors often participate by informally talking about the cultural conduct or customs of the group. They become active collaborators in the research rather than passive respondents. Key informants may be other health professionals or patients. DeSantis (1994) sees patients as the main cultural informants in nursing ethnography. They tell the nurses of their culture or subculture and of the expectations and health beliefs that form part of it.(Holloway & Wheeler , 1996).

Here is an example using key informant:. Key informant interviews were conducted for the health care providers and for a defaulter patient. Interviewing such individuals was a direct way of knowing as to how they, as well as the community they lived in, had perceived the content of information that was provided by the Information, Education And Communication (IEC) messages. For Key informant interviews, the four informants consisted of two private practitioners, one each from the walled city and slum area; one Anganwadi worker from a re-settlement colony and one defaulter patient who had been randomly picked by the team of investigators during their survey of the selected study settlement. (Ingle, Nath, Sharma & Taneja, 2008)

From the above mentioned study, the researcher initially desired to interview individuals with a broad knowledge about the concept or those who meet general criterions. As the study progresses, sample needs may change somewhat and selection criteria may be altered. Purposive sampling may evolve into theoretical sampling, which involves selecting participants or data sources that will contribute to the emerging theory (Jeanfreau and Leonard, 2010). It is therefore preferable to employ "theoretical" sampling of small numbers of people chosen for their special attributes. (Hollway, 1989; Charmaz, 1990; Miller & Crabtree, 1994; Yardley, 1997)

Theoretical sampling is another important type of purposive sample and is often used as part of a grounded theory approach to research. Glaser and Strauss (1967) define theoretical sampling as the process of data collection for generating theory whereby the analyst jointly collects, codes and analyzes his data and decides what data to collect next and where to find them in order to develop the…theory as it emerges. The researcher decides who or what to sample next, based on prior data gathered from the same research project in order to make comparisons with previous findings (Hesse-Biber & Leavy, 2006). So the Aanalyses of findings in our current analysis of the data and the theoretical insights we come up with provide us with new sampling questions like: Who will I talk with next? (The Practice Of Qualitative Research)

Mason (1996) said that theoretical sampling means selecting groups or categories to study on the basis of their relevance to our research questions, our theoretical position…and most importantly the explanation or account which we are developing. This theoretically-defined universe will make some sampling choices more sensible and meaningful than others. Mason describes choosing a kind of sample which can represent a wider population. (Mason, 1996; Silverman, 2005)

Theoretical sampling may be used in grounded theory. Theoretical sampling in grounded theory involves selecting participants who are capable of providing insight into emerging theoretical constructs (Collingridge and Gantt, 2008). Unlike other sampling which is planned beforehand, theoretical sampling in grounded theory continues throughout the study and is not planned before the study starts. In the view of Holloway & Wheeler (1996), 'At the start of the project, researchers make initial sampling decisions. They decide on a setting and on particular individuals or groups of people able to give information on the topic under study. Once the research has started and initial data hasve been analyzed and examined, new concepts arise,... people are chosen who can further illuminate the problem. Researchers then set out to sample different situations. Individuals...and focus on new ideas to extend the emerging theories. The selection of participants is a function of developing theories. Theoretical sampling continues until the point of saturation'. Here is another example. The data of this study is acquired from several villages in the rural area of Charghat Thana of Rajshahi district, Bangladesh by using a purposive sampling technique. Cox (1970) discovered the logistic regression model that can be used not only to identify risk factors but also to predict the probability of success. Furthermore, Lee (1980) and Fox (1984) developed this model. This model expresses a qualitative dependent variable as a function of several explanatory variables. Respondent's age, age at marriage, birth order, birth interval, household condition, sources of drinking water and breastfeeding are considered as explanatory variables in this model. We can find that the researchers involve selecting participants who are capable of providing insight into emerging theoretical constructs.

3) Qualities of good informants

Morse (1991) identifies the good informant: 'Good informants must be willing and able to critically examine the experience and their response to the situation...must be willing to share the experience with the interviewer'. Burgess (1985) also said that good informants who are especially sensitive to the area of concern and informants who are willing to discuss situations.

A good informant is one who is able to reflect and provide detailed experiential information about the phenomenon. And they must be willing and able to critically examine the experience and their response to the situation. The second quality of a good informant is that he or she must be willing to share the experience with the interviewer. Third, the willingness to talk is also related to the interviewee having enough uninterrupted time for the interview and sufficient patience and tolerance to explain and answer the researcher's question.(Morse, 1991)

As for key informants, they can be a good informant. They should own special knowledge about the history and subculture of a group, about interaction processes in it and cultural rules, rituals and language. They should be able to help the researcher to become accepted in the culture and subculture (Holloway & Wheeler, 1996). Moreover, the key informant should be a research collaborator. The key informant can first answer questions and provides the explanations-what, when, who, why, and how (Schatzman & strauss, 1973). The key informant will be able to help transform the researcher's translations of the native culture into something with meaning in the researcher's own culture. (Gilchrist, 1992)

Conclusion

Whom we talk to is crucial in qualitative design, so we should choose thoughtfully. All of the people that we interview should satisfy the requirements which are mentioned in the above sections. We should extend results from qualitative interviews and choose proper interviewees who can provide grounded and accurate information, talk enough with them to get a complete picture of the research area and feel confident that we understand it. Properly selecting informants can make good qualitythe qualitative research in a good quality.

Author's Background

Chung Tin Yu, Karen, a year two nursing student who is studying Master of Nursing in from The Hong Kong Polytechnic University and Hong Kong Sanatorium Hospital. (Email: 09696920g@polyu.edu.hk)

References

Biber S.N. & Leavy P. (2006). *The Practice Of Qualitative Research*. California: SAGE Publications.

Byrne M. (2001). *Sampling for qualitative research*. Retrieved November 24, 2010, form http://findarticles.com/p/articles/mi_m0FSL/is_2_73/ai_70871448/?tag=content;col1

Byington R. L., Grabner L. & Keene S. (2009). End Of Life Care For Latino Patients In Rural East Tennessee: Do Patients Believe Their Cultural Differences Are Important? . *The Internet Journal of World Health and Societal Politics*. Retrieved November 24, 2010, form http://www.ispub.com/journal/the_internet_journal_of_world_health_ and_societal_politics/volume_6_number_1_33/article/end_of_life_care_for_latino_p atients_in_rural_east_tennessee_do_patients_believe_their_cultural_differences_are_ important.html#h1-2

Collingridge D.S. & Gantt E.E. (2008). The Quality of Qualitative Research. *American Journal of Medical Quality*. Retrieved November 24, 2010, form http://ajm.sagepub.com.ezproxy.lb.polyu.edu.hk/content/23/5/389.full.pdf+html

DeSantis (1994). Ethnography. In Holloway I. & Wheeler S., *Qualitative Research For Nurses* (pp. 81-97). Cambridge: Blackwell Science

Finch J. & Mason J. (1990). Decision Taking in the Fieldwork Process: Theorettical Sampling and Collaborative Work. In Bryman A. & Burgess R. (Eds.), *Qualitative Research 1* (pp. 291-318). California: SAGE Publications.

Gilchrist V.J. (1992). Key Informant Interview. In Bryman A. & Burgess R. (Eds.), *Qualitative Research 1* (pp. 354-371). California: SAGE Publications.

Gobo G. (2004). Sampling, representativeness and generalizability. In Gobo G., Gubrium, Seale C. & Silverman D. (Eds.), *Qualitative Research Practice* (pp.435-456). California: SAGE Publications.

Goetz & LeCompte (1984). Ethnography. In Holloway I. & Wheeler S., *Qualitative Research For Nurses* (pp. 81-97). Cambridge: Blackwell Science

Glaser & Strauss (1967). The Research Process. In Biber S.N. & Leavy P. (Eds.), *The Practice Of Qualitative Research* (pp. 45-82). California: SAGE Publications.

Hossain M. & Islam M. R. (2009). Effects Of Demographic And Household Variables On Infants And Children Under -5five Mortality: An Application Of Logistic Model . *The Internet Journal of Health*. Retrieved November 24, 2010, form http://www.ispub.com/journal/the_internet_journal_of_health/volume_8_number_2_ 12/article/effects_of_demographic_and_household_variables_on_infant_and_child_u nder_five_mortality_an_application_of_logistic_model.html#h1-1

Holloway I. & Wheeler S. (1996). *Qualitative Research For Nurses*. Cambridge: Blackwell Science

Jeanfreau S.G.& Leonard J.J. (2010). *Appraising Qualitative Research in Health Education: Guidelines for Public Health Educators*. Retrieved November 24, 2010, form http://hpp.sagepub.com.ezproxy.lb.polyu.edu.hk/content/11/5/612.full.pdf+html

Leininger (1985). Ethnography. In Holloway I. & Wheeler S., *Qualitative Research For Nurses* (pp. 81-97). Cambridge: Blackwell Science

Mason (1996). Selecting a Case. In Silverman D. (Ed.), *Doing Qualitative Research* (pp. 125-138). California: SAGE Publications.

Morse J. M. (1991). *Qualitative Nursing research: A Contemporary Dialogue*. California: SAGE Publications.

Morse (1995). The Research Process. In Biber S.N. & Leavy P. (Eds.), *The Practice Of Qualitative Research* (pp. 45-82). California: SAGE Publications.

Nath A., Ingle G. K., Sharma N. & Taneja D. K. (2008). A Qualitative Evaluation Of The Information, Education And Communication (IEC) Component Of The Tuberculosis Control Programme In Delhi, India . *The Internet Journal of Tropical Medicine*. Retrieved November 24, 2010, form http://www.ispub.com/journal/the_internet_journal_of_tropical_medicine/volume_4_ number_2_47/article/a_qualitative_evaluation_of_the_information_education_and_c ommunication_iec_component_of_the_tuberculosis_control_programme_in_delhi_in dia.html

Rubin H.J. & Rubin I. S. (1995).*Qualitative Interviewing-The Art of Hearing Data*. California: sage Publications.

Schatzman & Strauss (1973). Key Informant Interview. In Bryman A. & Burgess R. (Eds.), *Qualitative Research 1* (pp. 354-371). California: SAGE Publications.

Yardley L. (1997). Dilemmas in Qualitative Health Research. In Bryman A. (Ed.), *Qualitative Research 2* (pp. 73-91). California: SAGE Publications.

In: Nursing Research: A Chinese Perspective   ISBN: 978-1-61209-833-3
Editor: Zenobia C. Y. Chan   ©2011 Nova Science Publishers, Inc.

Chapter XX

Can Qualitative Research Generalize?

H. Y. Tse and Zenobia C. Y. Chan
The Hong Kong Polytechnic University, China

Summary

Qualitative research is an objective and systematic approach to explore attitudes, behaviors and experiences via personal interviews or focus groups. These methods only consist of a small sample size. Qualitative research is commonly used in nursing to understand patients care. This paper focuses on whether qualitative research can generalize. Generalizability refers to applying a result from one sample to another sample. Philosophies of both quantitative and qualitative research arend discussed because the issue of generalizability should be traced back to the fundamental issues. Under the scope of the qualitative research, generalizing from a sample to a population is not the first priority. Instead it provides ways to understand human beings and social phenomenon. Since generalizability is rooted from the quantitative research, naturalists argue that it is inappropriate to evaluate the qualitative findings by generalizability. Other naturalists suggest that using transferability to evaluate whether one finding can be used in another population. Transferability is similar to generalizability but requires thick descriptions of the qualitative research. Thick descriptions include clear details of research design, site, sampling, data collection and data analysis method. A paper is evaluated in terms of the transferability, which demonstrates the generalizing power of a qualitative research.

Introduction

Qualitative research has long been cursed of its inability to generalize. This argument weakens the strength of the qualitative research and makes the qualitative research pointless and meaningless. It is therefore interesting and also a must for all qualitative researchers to look at the issue of generalizability before carrying on their work. Otherwise, all the efforts are in vain. In the essay, I will first reveal the concepts of both qualitative and quantitative research and generalizability. It's crucial to look back at the fundamentals before reviewing any in-depth arguments. Secondly, I will look at how positivists oppose the qualitative research in terms of the generalizability. Thirdly, I will discuss how qualitative researchers perceive the generalizability issue, and its ability to generalize from one setting to another by clearly re-defininge the concept of generalizability into transferability. The Ccondition of transferability is further explained. Lastly, a paper published by Journal of Clinical Nursing is used to demonstrate the use of transferability.

Overview of Quantitative Research and Qualitative Research

Research is gradually important in the nursing field to improve the quality of care. The two major methodologies are the quantitative research and qualitative research. They have their own aims and characteristics, respectively. Quantitative research uses empirical methods which take into account for the subjectivity and value neutrality. It measures the variables and produces figures which allow judgments (Sarantakos, 2005). On the other hand, qualitative research aims to produce insights on the social world, within natural settings, by giving meanings, experiences, practices and views of those involved (Craig and Smyth, 2007). It provides "thick descriptions" to describe, analyze and interpret (Holloway and Wheeler, 2010).

Nursing is a lovely mixture of pure science and social science. From a scientific perspective, nurses evaluate outcomes of the nursing interventions objectively. Quantitative research can do the favor. Interestingly, nurses provide care to human beings. Understanding human beings assists understanding nursing phenomenon, and qualitative research cannot be omitted. The quantitative research traditionally plays a dominant role in medical science but qualitative research is giving a remarkable contribution recently (Giacomini & Cook, 2004). It is believed that qualitative research is helpful in discovering the essence of nursing care.

What is Generalizability?

Generalizability is a criterion to evaluate the quantitative research. According to Campbell and Stanley (1963), 'External validity asks the question of generalizability: To what populations, settings, treatment variables, and measurement variables can the effect be generalized?' Generalizability refers to applying a research result from a sample to a population, and also across the populations (Babbie, 2010). Quantitative researcher's goal is to generalize results to diverse populations and times (Smith, 1975). Generalizability is based on the use of probability statistics. By simply selecting a random sample from the population, probability is calculated to judge whether the sample is representative (Sharp, 1998). Sampling is indispensable when using quantitative research. In nursing, researchers seek better interventions for patients to improve health outcome. If it is found that an intervention is useful in United States cancer patients, it is concluded that the intervention can be applied to elsewhere, such as Hong Kong. Only by the support of generalizability could it make research useful and widespread.

Opposing Qualitative Research by Generalizability

Probability sampling is the base of the quantitative research. However, qualitative research researchers often conduct qualitative interviewing, focus groups and observations to collect data (Babbie, 2010). They immerse themselves as a participant to understand the meaning of totality of the phenomenon (Dempsey & Dempsey, 2000). The researchers select a small sample and study thoroughly. Different perspectives are studied to understand social phenomenon.

Positivists blame that the case study is not consistent with the statistical sampling procedures. Based on the sampling and probability theory, if the sample is drawn randomly from a population, each member has an equal opportunity of falling in. The sampling theory can be used to predict how closely the sample represents the population by confidence interval which is the range around the sample value within which the population value will fall with a given probability (Firestone, 1993). However, qualitative researchers do not pick up the sample randomly but purposely. Positivists blame that the qualitative research finding cannot represent the whole population and its implication is meaningless. The lack of generalizability is cited as a major weakness of the qualitative research (Bolgar, 1965; Shaughnessy & Zechmeister, 1985).

It is interesting to see the criticism over the generalizability of the qualitative research but qualitative research is growing popularity, no matter in social science, education, nursing and medical. I truly believe that there must be some misconceptions of interpreting the generalizability in the qualitative research. Since generalizability is an indispensable element to evaluate the quantitative research, it is important to make the concept clear in the qualitative research. If generlizability is in appropriate in qualitative research, we should identify the essence of evaluating qualitative research. If a qualitative researcher cannot justify that, the previous work is meaningless.

What do Qualitative Researchers think?

There are different views towards generalizability in the qualitative field, namely ignorance, rejection and transferability.

Ignorance

Traditionally, the methodological literature on qualitative research has shown a little attention to the generalizability (Schofield, 1993). It is formidable to find out concepts related to generalizability in the textbooks. For example, in the Practice of Social Research written by Babbie (2010), the author only discussed the validity and reliability as the criteria to evaluate the qualitative research field. It is a shared view that the generalizability is unimportant or unachievable among qualitative methodological literature (Schofield, 1993). Personally, I do not think it is a good approach to avoid addressing the generalizability in qualitative research.

As generalizability is important in quantitative research, there is a need to mention it from the view point of qualitative research no matter it is achievable or not. Therefore, the following section is going to discuss others' views.

Rejection

The second view is rejecting the generalizability in qualitative research. Qualitative researchers do not regard generalization as their goal when conducting their research. They are not interested in sampling and probability theory and do not wish to generalize from a sample to population. The interpretivists interpret every instance of social interaction, if thickly described (Geertz, 1973) as a slice from the life world. Every single social interaction is a proper subject matter for them because it carries its own logic, sense of order, structure and meaning (Denzin, 1983).

Based on the philosophy of the qualitative research, some argue that it is inappropriate to fit generalizability into the research. The concept of generalizability in fact, violates the philosophy, purpose and intent of the qualitative paradigm. Under qualitative paradigm, the research aims to discover in-depth meanings, understandings and quality attributes of the phenomenon. It does not aim to provide the quantified outcomes. Leininger (1994) argue that the genralizability is inconsistent with the philosophy, purposes, and goals of qualitative paradigm and reduces the creditability of the findings. If one qualitative researcher tries to prove his research in terms of generalizability, it reflects his lack of knowledge and can be shameful. Personally, I think the qualitative research can be generalized depending on the objective sampling strategy. If a deviated case is selected, it is inappropriate tois generalize. If the general social process is studied, the qualitative research can generalize with caution.

Transferability

Why the caution has been taken? Cultural difference exists in different social phenomenon and generalizing from a population to another blindly is impossible. In qualitative research, cultural diversity and generalizability are like two opposing forces on the balance. Researchers want to investigate into the equilibrium between generalizing to another population and maintaining cultural uniqueness. In addition, direct application is impossible under qualitative paradigm due to the absence of probability sampling. Lastly, rejection of generalizability directs other methods for evaluation.

Goetz and LeCompte (1984) raised a term called "comparability" and "translatability" to put emphasis on the clear and detailed description. By analyzing the degree of differences from one situation to another, one is able to find out if the finding can generalize or not. These concepts allow extending one finding to other situations.

Many qualitative researchers suggest transferability as an alternative to generalizability (Auerbach & Silverstein, 2003). Transferability requires identifying both similarities and differences among the research and a new setting. It helps judge whether the contents of findings can transfer outside the study situation (Craig & Smyth, 2007). Although the theory derived from qualitative research is not universally applicable, the implication can be transferred in similar settings. We, therefore, have to understand the settings well before any transfer. Researchers have the responsibilities to provide adequate descriptive details. Readers can evaluate the transferability of qualitative research by looking at the "thick description". Thick descriptions include the site selection, sampling theory, instrument tool, data collection, storage and analysis method (Craig & Smyth, 2007). The more the details that are given, the easier the reader can judge whether the finding is transferable to their case. In addition, transferability serves as a method for others to imitate and study a new sample. When one applies a finding to a new sample, it is possible to understand the subjective experiences of those participants. Also, since different samples or groups or populations haves its own culture character, the researcher can extend the meanings and explore the theory further and deeper. Later on, a theory is defined by including perspectives from different samples (Auerbach & Silverstein, 2003).

Ignoring the issue of generalizability is not an appropriate choice. As a matter of fact, the abovementioned "comparability", "translatiability" and "transferability" make good use of generalizability. These concepts suggest providing thick descriptions to further enhance the implication of qualitative research findings. Readers compare theirhis own setting with the research setting to decide whether it is transferable or not. It is left upon the reader's judgement

Example of Transferability

I will utilize the concept of transferability to confirm whether it is practical to generalize findings from qualitative research. "Menstrual and menarche experience among pubescent female students in Taiwan: implications for health education and promotion practice" researched by Chang, Chen, Hayter and Lin was used. It was published in Journal of Clinical Nursing in 2008. The study aims to explore the menarche and menstruation experiences of young females in elementary education in Taiwan and provides clinical implication. The thick descriptions are evaluated in terms of the site selection and sampling strategy, data collection and data analysis method.

a)   Site selection and sampling strategy

According to the journal, the research was done in an elementary school in Hualien in Taiwan. A purposive sampling is used. The study recruited 20 female elementary students at their age of 10 to 12. Participant characteristics including age, menarche age, race and living status were given. Some participants lived with parents and some did not. All participants did not receive any menstrual education prior to their menarche.

The site was clearly given which enabled readers to judge whether the result is transferable. Cultural difference is a concern. As the sample was taken from Taiwan, the result may not be applicable in Britain. However, the finding may be transferable to Hong Kong due to the cultural similarity. Also, the demographic information was given. The Rreader can compare the research group and their own group before using the finding.

b)   Data collection method

Researchers used the focus group interviews as a data collection method. They assigned the participants into 3 groups. Each group consisted of six to eight participants. The semi-structured schedule was developed from the recent literature and the Guidelines for Pediatric Focus Group Research suggested by Heary and Hennessy (2002). The schedule provided open-ended questions to explore participants' views of menarche and menstruation from a biopsycholsocial perspective. Research team members facilitated the discussion and tape recorded it down and transcribed it verbatim for analysis. Filed notes were also taken during discussions to capture the key issues.

Permission was obtained from the appropriate school authorities. Information sheets and informed consent were given to the participants and their parents. Data confidentiality was ensured by coding participant information and transcripts. Data were anonymizedannoymised during transcription.

The researchers clearly described how to prepare and conduct the data collection method, including the focus group questions and ethical issues. Other researchers are able to imitate the study easily by following the thick descriptions. When the study is conducted in another sample, the theory can be well constructed.

c)   Data analysis method

The transcripts were analyzed by Atlas V5.0 software. Thematic analysis by Uskul (2004) and Joffe and Yardley (2004) were used. The researchers analyzed the menstrual experiences by three aspects, namely the physical effects, emotional issues and social dimension. Direct quotations of participants were included in the report according to each aspect.

The software and theoretical analysis provided adequate information for others to replicate the other's findings. Due to the culture diversity, researchers from different regions can replicate the study and discover new meanings of the menstural experiences.

Given the concept of transferability, one is able to compare the similarities and differences between the research and the current situation. The underpinning philosophy of qualitative research helps us to understand the meanings of human behavior and social phenomenon. The Rreader can transfer the implications from a qualitative research to a practical clinic area. It is left upon the reader's judgement based on the thick descriptions.

Conclusion

Generalizability, or more appropriately, transferability is acting in qualitative research and remains its strength. It is used depending on the study purpose. If the study wishes to provide meanings and interpretations for a population, it is essential for a researcher to provide thick descriptions. As a matter of fact, research has the duty to provide the detailed information with confidentiality regarding the ethical issues. In review of the literature, there is a lack of organized guidelines on how to evaluate the transferability. The current information is scattered. Researchers can enhance the qualitative research by working on a more comprehensive on guidelines of generalizability.

Author's Background

Tse Hei Yin, Constance Hei Yin Tse is studying the Master of Nursing in The Hong Kong Polytechnic University, after her bachelor in business management. Her goal is to pursue high quality of nursing care for the life time. (Email: heiyin98@gmail.com).

References

Auerbach, C. F., & Silverstein, L. B. (2003). *Qualitative data: an introduction to coding and analysis.* New York: New York University Press.

Babbie, E. (2010). The practice of social research. *U.S.A.*: Wadsworth Cengage Learning.

Bolgar, H. (1965). The case study method. In B.B. Wolman (Ed.), *Handbook of Clinical Psychology.* (pp. 28-39). New York: McGraw-Hill.

Campbell, D. & Stanley. J. (1963). "Experimental and quasi-experimental designs for research on teaching. In N. Gage (Ed.), *Handbook of research on teaching* (pp. 49-67). Chicago: Rand McNally.

Chang Y. T., Chen Y. C., Hayter M., & Lin M. L. (2009). Menstrual and menarche experience among pubescent female students in Taiwan: implications for health education and promotion practice, *Journal of Clinical Nursing, 18,* 2040-2048.

Craig, J. V., & Smyth, R. L. (2007). *The evidence-based practice manual for nurses.* Philadelphia: Elsevier Limited.

Dempsey, P. A., & Dempsey, A. D. (2000). Using nursing research process, critical evaluation, and utilization. *U.S.A.*: Lippincott Wiliams & Wilikins.

Denzin, N. K. (1983). Interpretive interactionism. In G. Morgan (Ed.), *Beyond method: strategies for social research* (pp. 129-146). Beverly Hills, CA: Sage.

Firestone, W. A. (1993). Alternative arguments for generalizaing from data as applied to qualitative research. *Educational Researcher, 22,* 16-23.

Geertz, C. (1973). Thick description: toward an interpretive theory of culture. In C. Geertz (Ed.), *The interpretation of cultures* (pp. 3-30). New York: Basic Books.

Giacomini, M. K., & Cook D. J. (2000). User's guide to the medical literature: XXIII. Qualitative research in health care A. Are the results of the study valid? *JAMA, 284* (3), 357-362.

Goetz, J. P., & LeCompte, M. D. (1984). *Ethnography and qualitative design in educational research.* Orlando, FL: Academic Press.

Heary, C. M., & Hennessy, E. (2002). The use of focus group interviews in pediatric health care research. *Journal of Pediatric Psychology, 27,* 47-57.

Holloway, I., & Wheeler, S. (2010). *Qualitative research in nursing and healthcare.* Malaysia: John Wiley & Sons.

Joffe, H. & Yardley, L. (2004). Content and thematic analysis. In D. F. Marks and L. Yardley (ed.), *Research methods for clinical and health psychology* (pp. 56-68). London: Sage.

Leininger, M. (1994). Evaluation criteria and critique of qualitative research studies. In J. M. Morse (ed.), *Critical issues in qualitative research methods* (pp. 95-116). California: Sage.

Sarantakos, S. (2005). *Social research.* New York: Palgrave MacMillan.

Schofield, J. W. (1993) Increasing the generalizability of qualitative research. In M. Hammersley (Ed.), *Social research: philosophy, politics and practice* (pp. 200-225). London: Sage.

Sharp, K. (1998). The case for case studies in nursing research: the problem of generalization. *Journal of Advanced Nursing, 27,* 785-789.

Shaughnessy, J. J., & Zechmeister, E. B. (1985) *Research methods in psychology.* New York: Knopf.

Smith, H. W. (1975). *Strategies of social research: the methodological imagination.* Englewood Cliffs, NJ: Prentice-Hall.

Uskul, A. K. (2004). Women's menarche stories from a multi-cultural sample. *Social Science and Medicine, 59,* 667 – 679.

In: Nursing Research: A Chinese Perspective
Editor: Zenobia C. Y. Chan

ISBN: 978-1-61209-833-3
©2011 Nova Science Publishers, Inc.

Chapter XXI

Qualitative Research: Credibility in Trustworthiness

W. Y. Yu and Zenobia C. Y. Chan
The Hong Kong Polytechnic University, China

Summary

Qualitative research is a method of inquiry to gather an in-depth understanding of human behavior and reasons governed by the researcher's interpretation. It is traditionally used in social science, and is increasingly recognized and valued in its unique place in nursing disciplines as highlighted by many. With the continuous raising of the problems of objectivity and the validity of qualitative research, this paper aims to focus on technical rigour: the researcher's role in maintaining credibility in trustworthiness. The role of the researcher influences on the internal validity (credibility) in qualitative research in several areas. Both diverse philosophical belief values of qualitative einquiry, as well as different roles of researchers during the research process will be discussed in detail. Finally, recommendations for researchers are suggested in order to provide a guide for them to conduct trustworthiness research papers in the future.

Introduction

Qualitative research aims to study the participant's viewpoint in order to understand the meaning of the totality of the phenomenon (Mason, 1996). Trustworthiness and rigour has an important role in all research processes, in the qualitative ones, the role of the researcher may alters a lot in maintaining its credibility. To sustain trustworthiness and rigour is clearly the key to successful researches since the result will be scientific evidence to be integrated into our knowledge base (Morse & Barrett, 2002; Long & Johnson, 2000). Thus, it is essential to investigate the roles and the competences of the researcher in the qualitative research in order to increase the trustworthiness in the credibility aspects. An overview of the importance of the researcher's role in the rigour and the key concepts of credibility issues in qualitative inquiry elements will be examined. In order to accomplish this, different roles of researchers in the qualitative research process will be evaluated in detail. Lastly, the paper ends with the recommendations for researchers to enhance the rigour and trustworthiness in the future research.

Trustworthiness and Rigour of Qualitative Research

Qualitative researches are detailed descriptions of situations, events, people, and interactions, observed behaviors, direct questions from people about their experiences, attitudes, beliefs, and thoughts and excerpts or entire passages from documents, correspondence, records, and case histories (Polit & Hungler, 1997). From the definition stated, it is believed that the qualitative research is not restricted to a set of methods or the nature of evidence. Although there is a proliferation of qualitative researches in the past several decades in advanced of the science of nursing as well as the collective understanding of the human health experience, it's always a difficulty toin judgeing the quality of qualitative research. Many researches point out that the positivist concepts of internal and external validity, reliability and objectivity do not translate into the qualitative paradigm. Therefore, most frequent criticisms directed at qualitative research are sloppy, *'merely subjective'* and above all, lacks rigour (Lincoln & Guba, 1985).

In facing the challenges of the current dialogue of the difficulty in establishing validity criteria in qualitative research, Lincoln and Guba (1985) propose four alternative measures to demonstrate its trustworthiness: *'credibility'*, *'transferability'*, *'dependability'* and *'confirmability'*. In this paper, the credibility will be the focused to of an in-depth analysis. Since the qualitative researcher is often cast as the "instructment" of data impinges on those data processes and are "part of the data" (Patton, 1990)., bBy exploring the researcher's role, it is believed that the aspects altering the trustworthiness and rigour of qualitative research can be investigated.

Principal Positions of Credibility Establishment

Credibility refers to the internal validity in qualitative research, which is the accuracy of the description of the phenomenon under investigation (Mays & Pope, 1995). The criterion involves establishing research results which are credible or believable from the perspective of the participant in the research. Philosophical belief in qualitative inquiry is a fundamental appreciation of naturalistic inquiry, qualitative methods, inductive analysis, purposeful sampling, and holistic thinking (Long & Johnson, 2000). With the rationale for, appreciation of, and worthwhileness of holistic thinking-all core paradigm themes; both scientists and non-scientists often hold strong opinions about what constitutes credible evidence. Given the potentially controversial nature of methods decisions, researchers using qualitative methods need to be prepared to explain and defend the value and appropriateness of qualitative approaches.

Apart from philosophical beliefs, rigorous techniques and methods for gathering high-quality data needed to be carefully recognized. Qualitative analysis is a creative process, depending on the insights and conceptual capabilities of the analyst (Munhall, 2001). More generally, beyond the analyst's preparation and creative insight, there is also a technical side to analysis that is analytically rigorous, mentally replicable, and explicitly systematic. Thus, this implies that, as a qualitative researcher, he or she has an obligation to be methodical in reporting sufficient details of data collection and the processes of analysis to permit others to judge the quality of the results. The main criterion depends on the researchers' training, experience, track record, status, and presentation of the research findings, which can in turn, alter the credibility in the research.

Researchers' Role in Credibility

Human behavior is greatly influenced by the external circumstances, including all of the settings, such as the performance of the researchers. Thus, the researcher, as human instruments in the qualitative research, can principally affect the final creditability or accuracy of the results. According to Hewitt (2007), there are four ways in which the presence of the researcher, or the fact that an evaluation is taking place, can directly affect the findings.

1) Reactions of program participants and staff to the presence of the qualitative fieldworker;
2) Changes in the fieldworker (the measuring instrument) during the course of the data collection or analysis, that is, instrumentation effects;
3) The predispositions, selective perceptions, and/or biases of the qualitative researcher; and
4) Researcher incompetence (including lack of sufficient training or preparation).

The presence of researchers can certainly make a difference in the setting under study. The fact is because the data being collected may be created under much tension and anxiety exerted on the performances below par (Hewitt, 2007). In brief, the researcher has a responsibility to think about the problem, make a decision about how to handle it in the field. And then attempt to monitor observer effects and minimize this tension atmosphere. Another concern is about evaluator effects on the extent to which the predispositions or biases of the evaluator, which may affects data analysis and interpretations. The interpretive and social construction underpinnings of the phenomenological paradigm mean that data from and about humans inevitably represent some degree of perspective rather than absolute truth (Hewitt, 2007). Since the researchers can learn from their experiences and generate personal insights, by this means, they may make their objectivity suspect with subjective point of views.

Overview of Underlying Competences of a Researcher

In the belowsections below, several competencies including researchers' training, experience and preparation, neutrality and impartiality and rapport-building with participants will be investigated to indicate the effects on the role of the researcher in credibility.

Researcher Training, Experience and Preparation

Introductory psychology or sociology course teachlearns that human perception is highly selective (Mason, 1996). Subsequently, when looking at the same scene, design, or object, different people will see different things., iIt is highly dependent on their interests, biases, and backgrounds. In research on selective perception documents, the inadequacies of ordinary human observation and certainly doubt is cast is doubt on the internal validity of observation. Hence, observational methods require disciplined training and strict preparation. Training includes learning how to write descriptively; practicing the disciplined recording of field notes; knowing how to separate detail from trivia in order to achieve the former without being overwhelmed by the latter; and using rigorous methods to validate observations (Minichiello et al., 1995). Careful preparation for making observations is as important as disciplined training. Preparation refers to preparing the mind is to learn how to concentrate during the observation for the detail implication of the respondents' behavior. Gaining experiences from studying via previous researches and other experienced researchers' leads to pre-expose the potential matters in the research process. This further get prepares ones self in coping with problems during the process. To conclude, it is essential for the researchers to have the concentration on scientific eyes and ears and taste, touch, and smell mechanisms throughout the entire research process with experience to enhance the trustworthiness and rigour.

Neutrality and Impartiality

Another addressed part is through the notion of neutrality and impartiality, as stated by Erlandson (1993), the researcher or evaluator perceived as being interested in the people under study. The issue of bias in qualitative research is important, and it demands special attention and discussion in any qualitative research methods. Essentially, these are all concerns about the extent to which the qualitative researcher can be trusted in the methodological rigorour, such as reflecting the subjects and conditions during collecting and analyzing the data (Lincoln & Guba, 2000). Therefore, it is believed that the self of the researcher himself has an effect upon the subject and context of study. It starts from accepting the assumption until the attempt to control for the influence of the research process. And it is always an obligation for qualitative researchers to reflect the participants' viewpoint instead of over-reporting their subjective ideas in the research.

Rapport Building with Participants

Rapport- building between researchers and participants is crucial in relating to obtaining further in-depth data. A good rapport is essential to be established in the opening; with a cooperative and insightful participant (Jarman, 1995). Technique refers to the approaches the interviewer uses to keep an interview "on track." It includes skills to appropriately select questions in order to arrive at a therapeutically engagement with participants. From the beginning, the researchers have to show sensitivity to the participant's needs and lead to a forging a therapeutic alliance. Building on it, the researcher's targeted questions prove his or her understanding and expertise, which qualify him or her as a guide for the research. With the rapport- building, trust can be summated, and the trustworthiness of the data can be enhanced. In order to give a clear picture on how to build rapports in the research process, we will analyze the rapport- building in three different areas: personal, behavioral and cultural. According to MaCann & Haber (2001), the above three areas are the main areas where rapport can be built upon. Personal rapport is a participant's beliefs about themselves and the world must be totally accepted. The researchers must assume that what the participants said is the truth and to build on their model of the world to help them move themselves on to a more empowering belief. The next rapport-building is by building behavioral rapport, which is to match all the nuances of behavior that a participant exhibits. The physiological, tonal and language are the areas that should be focused on in order to synchronize with the pace of the participants. Building cultural rapport is to demonstrate the understanding and appreciation of the participant's culture through demonstrating the knowledge, showing or respecting certain behavior or using specific language common to that culture. By analyzing three different areas in rapport- building, it is believed that this is a process of building a sustaining relationship of mutual trust, harmony and understanding. And rRapport is the key to influence by starting with acceptance of the other person's point of view, their state and their style of communication.

With all of the underlying competences discussed above, we will explore different roles of the researcher in the entire research process in advanced, to provide a profound guide for the researcher to conduct a trustworthyiness and rigourous research.

Different Roles of Researchers in the Qualitative Research Process

In the following parts, we will explore the functions and roles of the researcher in four stages, comprisinges of the initial stage of participant recruitment, data collection, data analysis and production of the report and validation.

In the initial stage of participants' recruitment, control over the research process lays in the hands of the researcher, who decides the introduction of the research to potential participants, description of the research goals, and disclosure of institutional affiliations to enlist maximum cooperation (Bravo-Moreno, 2003). The amount and quality of the information offered regarding the research are entirely at the researcher's discretion andts to participate in the research and share their personal experience and knowledge. The dependence of the researcher on the participants' consent might enable participants to obtain more information about the research and the researcher (Mantzoukas, 2004). Therefore, at this stage, ethical dilemmas involve questions about strategically obscuring some of the research goals to persuade the participants to take part in the study..

For the researcher's' role in the data collection stage, it seems to be entirely dependent on the participants' willingness to take part in the research and to share their knowledge of the research subject with the researcher (Brinkmann & Kvale, 2005). At this stage, control and ownership of the data seem to be in the hands of the participants. The quantity and quality of the data shared with the researcher depends, in part, on the relationships that develops between the researcher and various participants, so rapport- building arises thein importance as mentioned above. The researcher must try to elicit the participants' stories as much as possible, their experiences, and their wealth of knowledge of the research topic. Achieving heightened empathy or informed consent using these methods is considered a process that is likely to increase participation and the richness of the research data (Kvale, 1996). The warm, caring, and empowering character of qualitative interviews is believed to conceal huge power differences, and the dialogue that takes place in the interviewing process might be a cover for the exercise of power in researches.

In the termination of the data collection stage, formal control and power over the data returns to the researcher. During the stage of data analysis and production of the report, the researcher's control over the data seems to be absolute and ethical considerations are of utmost importance. The researcher has total responsibility toward the participants, the research project, and the institution (Krayer, 2003). The decision to share varies according to the researcher's world view, qualitative research paradigm, and the nature of the research content. The researcher must ask themselvesf what additional knowledge will be gained from involving the participants in the analysis in order to have more valid and comprehensive data collected.

In the validation stage, after data collection and analysis are completed, some researchers choose to re-engage participants, with the objective of strengthening the trustworthiness, accuracy, and validity of the findings. The re-engagement is implemented through follow-up interviews meant to check the authenticity of emerging insights identified by researchers and verification of participants' intended meanings (Cutcliffe, 2000). Member checking is carried out individually or in a group, in which participants have the opportunity to discuss the findings and conclusions of the study (Hewitt, 2007). This process is meant to decrease the risk of misinterpretation of the participants' stories by providing inaccurate generalizations and hence, enhance the trustworthiness in the researches.

Recommendations for Researchers

Enhancement of the rigour and trustworthiness of participatory evaluations requires the use of methods, criteria and strategies that are appropriate to those involved in a particular research with the researchers' skills, knowledge and resources (Quinn, 1995). The ideal is that rigour is incorporated into all stages of the evaluation and that is closely related to the researchers' evaluation professionalism. By reviewing the above criteria and aspects, I have identified a number of strategies that can increase the rigour and trustworthiness of each stage in research and evaluation process. These strategies include community participation, engagement and communication methods can develop relations of mutual trust and open communication. Researchers should properly use of multiple theories and methodologies, multiple sources of data, and multiple methods of data collection. This can enhance an ongoing meta-evaluation and critical reflection with critical assessment of rigorous data analysis and reporting processes.

Conclusion

The paper examines the underlying competences and roles of the researcher in the research process; it is believed that the credibility of the research is controlled a lot in the hands of the researcher instead of the participants. As a researcher, he or she should expose to extensive training, experience and preparation to utilize the entire quality in the research process. Besides, researchers should have a perspective to be neutral and impartial in mind in order to maintain the credibility in qualitative research. And this can be further enhanced by the rapport- building between the researcher and the participants because more in-depth data and personal stories can be collected from the participants, thus productive and rich information can thus be collected.

In advanced research, there is a depth exploration on different roles in the research stages: initial participant recruitment, data collection, data analysis and production of the report and validation. This helps researchers to have a better understanding of their roles in sustaining the credibility during different stages. Whileith qualitative research has increasingly recognized its unique place in nursing disciplines, recommendations about the strategies to enhance rigour and trustworthiness are suggested to guide the further improvement and evaluation in the clinical research.

Author's Background

Yu Wing Yan, a year two student who is studying Master of Nursing in Hong Kong Polytechnic University and the Hong Kong Sanatorium Hospital. Having previous studies in Bachelor Degree of Hotel and Catering Management in Hong Kong Polytechnic University, the preservation of high quality care with evidence-based is highlighted. Nurses should have good preparation in all aspects, including the research competences toin fortify for the professional development. (Email: wingyanyuy@yahoo.com.hk)

References

Bravo-Moreno, A. (2003). Power games between the researcher and the participant in the social inquiry. *The Qualitative Report*, 8(4), 624-639.

Brinkmann, S., & Kvale, S. (2005). Confronting the ethics of qualitative research, *Journal of Constructivist Psychology*, 18(2), 157-181.

Cutcliffe, J. R. (2000). Methodological issues in grounded theory. *Journal of Advanced Nursing, 31*(6), 1476-1484.

Erlandson, D. A. (1993). *Doing a naturalistic inquiry: a guide to methods.* London: Sage.

Hewitt, J. (2007). Ethical components of researcher- researched relationships in qualitative interviewing. *Qualitative Health Research, 17,* 1149-1159.

Jarman, F. (1995). Communication problems: a patient's view. *Nursing Times, 91,* 30-31.

Krayer, A. (2003). Fieldwork, participation and practice: Ethics and dilemmas in qualitative research. *Sociology of Health and Illness, 25*(1), 134-136.

Kvale, S. (1996). *Interviews: An introduction to qualitative research interviewing.* London: Sage.

Lincoln, Y. S., & Guba, E. G. (1985). *Naturalistic Inquiry.* Newbury Park, CA: Sage.

Lincoln, Y. S., & Guba, E. G. (2000). Paradigmatic controversies, contradictions, and emerging confluences. *The handbook of qualitative research* (2nd ed.). Thousand Oaks, CA: Sage.

Long, T., & Johnson, M. (2000). Rigour, reliability and validity research. *Clinical Effectiveness in Nursing, 4*(1), 30–37.

MaCann, T. V., & Haber, H. (2001). Mutual relating: developing interpersonal relationships in the community. *Journal of Advanced Nursing, 34,* 530-537.

Mantzoukas, S. (2004). Issues of representation within qualitative inquiry. *Qualitative Health Research, 14,* 994-1007.

Mays, N., & Pope, C. (1995). Rigour and qualitative research. *British Medical Journal, 311,* 109–112.

Mason, J. (1996). *Qualitative Researching.* London: Sage.

Minichiello, V., Aroni, R., Timewell, E., & Alexander, L. (1995). *In-depth interviewing: Principles, techniques, analysis* (2nd ed.). Melbourne, Australia: Longman Cheshire.

Morse, J. M., & Barrett, M. (2002). Verification strategies for establishing reliability and validity in qualitative research. *International Journal of Qualitative Methods, 1*(2), 1–19.

Munhall, P. L. (2001). *Nursing Research: A Qualitative Perspective* (3rd ed.). MA: Jones and Bartlet.

Patton, M. Q. (1990). *Qualitative Evaluation and Research Methods.* Thousand Oaks, CA:Sage Publications.

Polit, D. F., & Hungler, B..P. (1997). *Essentials of Nursing Research.* Philadelphia: Lippincott.

Quinn, F. M. (1995). *The OPrinciples and Practice of Nurse Education* (3rd ed.). London: Chapman & Hall.

In: Nursing Research: A Chinese Perspective
Editor: Zenobia C. Y. Chan

ISBN: 978-1-61209-833-3
©2011 Nova Science Publishers, Inc.

Chapter XXII

Nursing Research Designs: Descriptive Correlational Design and Mixed Method Design

O. T. Li and Zenobia C. Y. Chan
The Hong Kong Polytechnic University, China

Summary

The significance of a correct research design and the elements of research design for a new researcher to consider when deciding the research approach for a specific study will be discussed in this paper. It is crucial for new researchers to have the above knowledge to maximize the validity of the study. The objective of the paper is to discuss and compare two research designs: descriptive correlational design and mixed method design. Research studies that are conducted using one of these research designs will be chosen as an example to demonstrate the purpose of choosing that particular design with the associated topic. Moreover, the advantages and disadvantages of the research design will be discussed.

Definition of a Good Research Design

A good research design can produce a significant outcome of a research study which can capture a group of audience's attention and lead to publication in well-recognized journals with further discussions or investigations on that subject (Huff, 2009). However, lots of researchers' works get rejected due to poor preparation for the study, such as choosing the wrong research design for their own purpose. Therefore, a suitable research design for the study can be a big stepping stone towards publication of the research work. As a result, it is crucial for new researchers to understand which research design suits well with their topics in order to have a convincing result for general recognition from the scholars.

Before going into more detailed about research design, it is essential to have a thorough understanding of what research design is. The term research design can be applied into two different situations: the process of recognizing the interest of study to the preparation for data collection or a 'defined structures within which the study is implemented' (Burns and Grove, 2001, p.223). A correct research design not only can satisfy the practical requirement but provide a deeper exploration of the topic; also, it can confirm and provide evidence of any existing conceptss or new discoveries of the topic (Huff, 2009). The selection criteria of a research design for study will be investigated below.

At the beginning of selecting the right research design, there are a few issues that should be addressed by the researcher: causality, bias, manipulation, control and validity. They are all closely related to each other for promoting strong rigor of the study. Causality is defined as the origin of the effect (Burns and Grove, 2001). In order to identify the causality of the subject, Houser (2008) suggests that researchers should identify the correlation of the possible independent variables and dependent variables such that there are no other alternative causations for the consequence. Then, the suspected cause and effect identified will have strong linksed between their existences to the event. Therefore, the researchers can focus on the variables which are more likely to give the possible explanation to the outcome of the phenomenon that they want to investigate.

Bias can occur when there is deliberate selection by researchers in any parts of the research design such as choosing participants without randomization (Miller and Yang, 2008). Hence, bias that is created by extraneous factors such as the investigator, the participants, the instrument used for investigation and other environmental factors can affect the evidence supporting the possible cause and the rigor of the study (Burns and Grove, 2001; Houser, 2008). If the research direction is towards an experimental design, manipulation of the variables should be considered and be carefully monitored to prevent any bias influencing the result (Burns and Grove, 2001). However, due to uncontrollable environment and ethical issues in nursing research, experimental design is hardly used (Gillis & Jackson, 2002). Therefore, researchers should constantly revise their research process to make sure bias is limited in the study and any uncontrolled variables appearing in the environment should be stated as the limitation for the research design.

Control is often used in quantitative studies for monitoring extraneous variables (Polit, Beck and Hungler, 2001). The stronger the ability to control the variables in the study, the more convincing of the study is (Burns and Grove, 2001). Therefore, a stronger relationship between the investigated variables will be identified (Miller and Yang, 2008). However, the more the extraneous variables are controlled in the study; the environment condition under the study is further fromless close to the real situation. As a result, the data collected may not be truly representing the reality. Thus, there is no control of extraneous variables in qualitative studies. On the other hand, for quantitative studies, control should be carefully adjusted to maintain the rigor of the study.

Bannigan and Watson (2009) define validity as 'the degree to which a scale measures what it is intended to measure' (p.3238). In addition, Whittemore, Chase and Mandle (2001) suggest that validity should be assessed according to the objective of the research topic. This is because validity in the study is the key for the development of investigation tools (Bannigan and Watson, 2009). Thus, Houser (2008) recommends that researchers should examine whether the description of the method has provided a full picture of the procedures of the investigation to the readers in the report. The method described can either be able to reproduce with a similar result using other subjects or be able to compare with other results from similar studies if the research is rigorous. Therefore, the validity of a research design plays a significant role in producing a good recognizable result for the study.

A good design should be 'rigorous and systematic' (p.186) and data collected from it should be convincing (Houser, 2008). It is difficult to choose the best research design to fit into the particular study. However, a relatively suitable research design can be chosen according to the research topic (Fitzpatrick, 1998). Oman, Krugman and Fink (2003) suggest that exploratory or descriptive research design can be used if the topic is not well studied in the past. Experiment or quasi-experiment design can be used alternatively when the investigated topic is previously explored. Hence, a comprehensive literature review for the topic is essential to deciding one a suitable research design.

Burns and Grove (2001) state that when a research question is chosen, there are criteria for choosing a good design which can enhance the likelihood of collecting good results. A good design should be able to serve the intention of the research, possibly set sensible limitations and successfully limit the possible bias which may endanger the validity of the study. Moreover, the design should be able to clearly deliver the focus of the study, the environment and the procedures such that they can be easily investigated by the others. The subjects of the study should be comparatively similar apart from the responses being evaluated. Furthermore, external variables in the environment may affect the data collection process. It would be best to recognize the external variables and restrict them from influencing any manipulations added during the study. If researchers follow the criteria mentioned above in deciding the research design, the rigor of the study can be strengthened and the results produced from the study can be more persuasive to the audience.

Research Designs used in Nursing

In nursing research, researchers often try to investigate perspectives of individuals, a particular incident or prodigy in clinical settings, therefore, exploratory, descriptive and epidemiologic, apart from experimental designs are often used (Oman, Krugman and Fink, 2003). This is because it is hard to control variables in clinical settings for experimental approach because it may violate the research ethics. By just describing the important issues needed to be addressed by the new researchers, ones may not fully understand what they should do for their research design. Therefore, in this paper, two methods used in nursing research, which are descriptive correlational design and mix-method designs, will be discussed below to illustrate how the design is implemented into the study. Moreover, the advantages and disadvantages of each research design will be discussed. In addition, examples of each research design will be given to illustrate the decision of using the particular design.

Definition and Characteristics of Correlational Study

Correlational study is a non-experimental research design which tries to investigate the linkage between different variables (Burns and Grove, 2001). Furthermore, it can be used when the independent variables cannot not be manipulated in the experimental study (Martin and Thompson, 2000). According to Omen and her colleagues (2003), the investigated variables should have a close association with each other in a ccorrelational study which helps to support the proposed arguments in the research. The information collected from the investigation will be in quantitative format which gives strong empirical evidence on the connection between the variables. However, the relationship between the variables is not necessary in a cause-and-effect relationship (Beins, 2004). Regarding the validity of the correlational study, the vigor of correlation coefficients should be acknowledged before the empirical examination of validity (McDowell and Newell, 1996). Therefore, the correlation coefficient in the study can influences the trustworthiness of the method used in correlational study.

Descriptive Correlational Design as a Type of Correlational Design

Descriptive correlational design is a type of correlational studyies which attempts to recognize and describe the variables without any interruption applieds to the environment (Burns and Grove, 2001). Therefore, it is able to examine the amount of intimacy between the variables and offer a platform for further experimental investigation in the future (Houser, 2008). However, it does not help to clarify or figure out the reasons of the linkage between the variables (Polit, Beck and Hungler, 2001). Hence, descriptive correlational design generally offers a descriptive relationship between the variables in the reality situation.

Bailey, Sabbagh, Loiselle, Boileau and McVey (2009) use a descriptive correlational study to investigate the relationships between three variables: family member's perception of informational support by the ICU nurses, anxiety level of family members and their satisfaction with nursing care. This design enables the researchers to describe the inter-relationships between variables. Three different forms of questionnaires are used to find out the score for each variable.

Test-retest method is used in this study as a control tool for the results obtained. This can ensure the data collected isare constantly reliable and stable (Fain, 2009). The order of the questionnaires is inspecting the anxiety level first, then satisfaction with care, perception of informational support and the socio-demographic information. In this way, the influence of the data obtained for the anxiety level will be diminished without concerning the following factors investigated therefore; the variation of variables obtained can be controlled (Bailey et al., 2009). Thus, Bailey and her colleagues have considered and identified different extraneous variables that can influence their data collection and try to minimize those extraneous variables to increase the rigor of the study.

From the results in this study, they are able to show a strong relationship between information support from nurses and satisfaction with care by the individuals. They conclude that the study provides a 'potentially meaningful "grass roots" initiative to improve the informational and psycholosocial care of family members of critically ill patients' (p.121) and suggest to have a larger scale of assessment such as quasi-experimental randomized clinical trail for this informational nursing practice (Bailey et al., 2009). This helps to show the aim of using descriptive correlational design in this study is to give background knowledge for the future study. However, this study does not provide the explanation of this phenomenon which is the drawback of descriptive correlational design.

In the study conducted by O'Haver, Melnyk, Mays, Kelly and Jacobson (2009), the insight of obesity verweight in adolescents is investigated. Few factors are taken into consideration regarding their relationships with obesity overweight, for instance, self-esteem, realization of being overweight, depression and anxiety. Descriptive correlational design is used to describe the relationship between those factors themselves. It is found that self-concept of attempting to lose weight is related to the BMI percentile (O'Haver et al., 2009). Moreover, the data is supported by other pervious studies. However, the data cannot be generalized since the sample size is small. Moreover, further reasons for such relationships is not able to be explained in this study.

To conclude the above two descriptive correlational studies, they both help to develop further experimental testing in the future which is one of the strengths about descriptive correlational design. Nevertheless, descriptive correlational studies are unable to identify the causation of each relationship. Moreover, each variable of interests may not show a correlation between each other which may lead to an unproductive research study. Therefore, it is important to address the linkage of possible variables before any investigation.

Definition and Characteristics of Mixed-Method Design

Mixed-method design has been recognized as involving qualitative and quantitative elements in investigating the research question. Mixed-methods can give a more complete perspective and knowledge of the study, refine explanation and give an in- depth look into the matter. Moreover, it enriches the explanation to the research question which leads to a greater support for the conclusion of the study (Johnson, Onwuegbuzie and Turner, 2007). Borkan (2004) proposes that mixed-method is able to assist researchers to investigate a more complicated event and they are able to approach the problem in a numerical and descriptive way. Thus, the phenomenon of interest can be better described and explained via mixed-method.

A mixed-method approach is used to give an extensive investigation of the degree of barriers and the influence of facilitators in response to the healthcare decision support from call center nurses (Stacey, Graham, O'Connor and Pomey, 2005). Surveys, interviews, focus groups and simulated patient calls are used to identify each factor influencing the decision support provided to the callers. This can provide further perceptions and approaches apart from using one method for the investigation (Borkan, 2004). Moreover, drawbacks of using a single method can be minimized (Polit and Beck, 2004). Although multi-methods are used, there are still 'non-response bias, reporting bias and generalizability beyond this single call center' (Stacey et al., 2005, p.192). Therefore, method triangulation does not necessary cover all the bias in the environment.

Although the bias cannot be completely eliminated, many factors which influences the outcome of decision- making can be identified using this method in the study, for instance, lack of decision- support, knowledge and techniques, organizational policies and resources provided for nurses limit the support nurses can provide to the callers (Stacey et al., 2005). However, new researchers who attempt to use a mixed-method design for their study should consider their amount of time they want to spend for data collection since multiple methods are used. Moreover, they have to be familiar with the different methods they use for the investigation because it can be very time- consuming and difficult to collect the expected results.

Another mixed-method study which is done by Schofield, Knussen and Tolson (2005) tries to explore the experiences of COPD patients and families regarding the health care services and care options. Relationships between patient's care options is strongly linked to the family's preference in this study. Survey and qualitative interviews are used in this study, trying to collect information in details. However, the data collected in both methods are retrospective which may affect the preciseness of the result. The questionnaire is adjusted according to the response collected after the pilot study; therefore, it enhances the accuracy of the responses in the main survey (Schofield et al., 2005). The result from the survey, which is about the choice of accepting treatment at home, echoes with the interview result. This strengthens the rigorousness of the performed study.

Comparing the method used for the two mixed-method studies above, the work of Schofield and her colleague is less time- consuming since there are only two interventions used for the investigation. Thus, researchers should adjust the type of method they want to use according to their time schedule if they decide to use mixed-method for their investigation.

Conclusion

It is important to choose the correct research design for the purpose of the study. Several factors such as causality, control, bias and validity should be considered while choosing the research design. By addressing the factors above, a good validity of the study can be established. However, there are always limitations that cannot be manipulated for the present research designs. It is difficult to find the best research design which fits all the criteria for the aim of a particular study. Therefore, researchers should be cautious and try to identify the limitations of the research design when they present their results for their studies.

Descriptive correlational design and mixed method design are discussed in this paper with examples shown to illustrate the reason for the choice of the design. Both designs have advantages and drawbacks for providing a good outcome for the study. It is important for researchers to address those limitations given by the design they have chosen for the research studies. Last but not the least, whether choosing descriptive correlational or mixed-method design for the study totally depends on the approach that the researcher wants to take to view the subject.

Author's Background

Li On Ting, Zoe Li, has graduated as a Bachelor of Medical Science student in University of Sydney, is continuing her further study in Master of Nursing in Hong Kong Polytechnic University. (Email: ontingli@hotmail.com)

References

Bailey J. J., Sabbagh M., Loiselle C. G., Boileau J. & McVey L. (2009) Supporting families in the ICU: a descriptive correlational study of informational support, anxiety, and satisfaction with care. *Intensive and Critical Care Nursing (2010)* 26, 114-122.

Bannigan K. & Watson R. (2009) Reliability and validity in a nutshell. *Journal of Clinical Nursing,* 18, 3237-3243.

Beins B. C. (2004) *Research methods: a tool for life.* United States of America: Pearson Education.

Borkan J. M. (2004) Mixed methods studies: a foundation for primary care research. *Annals of Family Medicine 2004*, 2:4-6.

Burns N. & Grove S. K. (2001) *The practice of nursing research: conduct, critique, & utilization.* (4th Ed) United States of America: W.B. Saunders company.

Fain J. A. (2009) *Reading, understanding, and applying nursing research.* (3rd Ed.) Philadelphia: F.A. Davis Co.

Fitzpatrick J. J. (1998) *Encyclopedia of nursing research.* United States of America: Springer Publishing Company.

Gillis A. & Jackson W. (2002) *Research for nurses: methods and interpretation.* Philadelphia: F. A. Davis Co.

Houser J. (2008) *Nursing research: reading, using, and creating evidence.* United States of America: Jones and Bartlett Publishers.

Huff A.S. (2009) *Designing research for publication.* United States of America: SAGE publications.

Johnson R. B., Onwuegbuzie A. J. & Turner L. A. (2007) Toward a definition of mixed methods research. *Journal of Mixed Methods Research April 2007*, 1(2): 112-133.

Martin C. R. & Thompson D. R. (2000) *Design and analysis of clinical nursing research studies.* London: Routledge.

McDowell I. & Newell C. (1996) *Measuring Health: a guide to rating scales and questionnaires* (2nd ed.) New York: Oxford University Press Inc.

Miller , G. J. , & Yang, K. (2008). HaHandbook *of research methods in public administration (2nd ed.).* Retrieved from http://www.crcnetbase.com.ezproxy.lb.polyu.edu.hk/ISBN/9780849353840

O'Haver J., Melnyk B. M., Mays M. Z., Kelly S. & Jacobson D. (2009) The relationship of perceived and actual weight in minority adolescents. *Journal of Pediatric Nursing December 2009*, 24(6): 474- 479.

Oman K. S., Krugman M. E. & Fink R. M. (2003) *Nursing research secrets.* United States: Hanley & Belfus.

Polit D. F. & Beck C. T. (2004) *Nursing research: principles and methods*. (7th Ed). United States of America: Lippincott Williams & Wilkins.

Polit D. F., Beck C. T. & Hungler B. P. (2001) *Essentials of nursing research: methods, appraisal, and utilization*. (5th Ed). United States of America: Lippincott Williams & Wilkins.

Schofield I., Knussen C. and Tolson D. (2006) A mixed method study to compare use and experience of hospital care and a nurse-led acute respiratory assessment service offering home care to people with an acute exacerbation of chronic obstructive pulmonary disease. *International Journal of Nursing Studies 2006*, 43: 465-476.

Stacey D., Graham I.D., O'Connor A. M. & Pomey M (2005) Barriers and facilitators influencing call center nurses' decision support for callers facing values-sensitive decisions: a mixed method study. *Worldviews on Evidence-Based Nursing 2005*, 2(4): 184-195.

Whittemore R., Chase S. K. & Mandle C. L. (2001) Validity in Qualitative research. *Qualitative health research July 2001*, 11(4): 522-537.

In: Nursing Research: A Chinese Perspective
Editor: Zenobia C. Y. Chan

ISBN: 978-1-61209-833-3
©2011 Nova Science Publishers, Inc.

Chapter XXIII

No Ethical Issue, No Clinical Research

Maggie K. Y. Lung and Zenobia C. Y. Chan

The Hong Kong Polytechnic University, China

Summary

Ethical issues are increasingly reviewed by different institutions across the world, with greater engagement with these processes occurring now (Council for International Organizations of Medical Sciences & World Health Organization, 2002; UNAIDS, 2007; World Medical Association, 2000). Conflicts between the goal of science and the need to protect rights and welfare of human research participants result in the center of ethical tension in clinical research (Derenzo & Moss, 2006); however, some other ethical issues addressing the integrity of clinical research should not be ignored. When even one part of a research project is questionable or conducted unethically, the integrity of the entire project is called into question (Derenzo & Moss, 2006). Thus, it is important for us to understand the rationale behind ethical principles in doing research. Based on the evidence of unethical research conducted in the past, this paper would outline different codes issued. Then some ethical principles required for clinical research would be discussed and would be followed by illustrations on the importance of addressing ethical issues properly and sincerely in clinical research. Although the paper would not cover all ethical issues or protocol sections, it aims to assist researchers doing clinical research to be more familiar with ethical considerations.

Introduction

Clinical research is defined as "the systematic collection of information from human and /or from organic material taken from humans to produce generalizable findings" (Derenzo & Moss, 2006, p.3). A clinical research allows researchers to look for a more effective method of care or treatment which benefits future patients (Derenzo and Moss, 2006). Although clinical research does not aim to anticipate benefits directly to the patients who participated, it is by no means that harm is done to anyone while the research is conducted. Therefore, it is most important that a clinical research is conducted in an ethically acceptable manner. In this paper, it would first define the term ethics. Second, some notable examples of unethical research conducted in the past would be illustrated and would be followed by the history of ethical research. Then, the principles of ethical research would be identified and the importance of ethics in clinical research would be discussed. Finally, the paper would conclude with reasons you have to address the ethical issue properly.

Ethics

Talbot and Perou (2001) defined ethics "as the discipline of describing behavior, practices, thinking and moral values generally agreed to be acceptable to society" (Talbot & Perou, 2001, p.63). In the broadest sense, ethics helps us answer how we ought to live and behave with reason (Grady, 2007). With respect to clinical research, we should ask ourselves whether it is necessary to do research on humans and how ethical principles of research should be put into practice to assure the research involving human subjects would be carried out in an ethical manner. Grady (2007) stated that "Through history, the perception and acceptance of methods, goals and scope off clinical research has shifted significantly along the attention to and appreciation of what respecting and protecting the human involved in the research entails" (p.16). This is coherent with the views that Aveyard and Hawley (2007) mentioned in that the term used to describe the human participating in the research changed from "subject" to "participant" illustrated that the researcher began to pay attention to the importance of the client's involvement and addressing their ethical rights. It is crucial to address the ethical issue in clinical research properly, ands if not, a number of consequences of conducting an unethical research would occur. The most notable example of unethical research conducted would be discussed to illustrate the need of addressing ethical issues properly and sincerely in clinical research.

Consequences of Conducting Unethical Research

In 1932, the Tuskegee Syphilis Study was conducted in Alabama for about 40 years by the U.S. Public Health Service to study the natural progression of untreated syphilis. The participants were given free medical exams, free meals and free burial insurance; however, their diagnosis of having syphilis was never told to them and the risks involved in the research were not disclosed. They were deceived to be treated for "bad blood" and left without treatment even though penicillin became a standard cure for syphilis in 1947 (Hesse-Biber & Leavy, 2006; Jones, 1993). As there were no voluntary consents, no previous investigation on the danger of the experiment on animals, and no proper medical protection and management, this study was unethical and put the integrity of the entire project into question. The experiment violated the ethical standard significantly by abusing the subject in which the individual was not just prone to harm but deaths, and gave a bad reputation towards the scientific community (Hesse-Biber & Leavy, 2006; Jones, 1993). With this unethical research being revealed, different guidelines and a code of ethics were issued to address the importance of ethical research. A brief introduction of the history of ethical issue in clinical research would outline the changes in demanding higher ethical concerns in conducting research.

History of Ethical issue in Clinical Research

Throughout history, there are several influential documents that have helped shape our sense of having ethical research. As stated by the University of Minnesota Center for Bioethics (2003), the birth of ethical research began with a desire to protect human subjects involved in research projects. The first code for human subject research is The Nuremberg Code, which was written in 1949 in response to Nazi experiments and raised the need forof voluntary consent of the subject. Then, the Declaration of Helsinki was developed in 1964 and having revised several times with the latest update occurring in 2000 to emphasize thate research should be of generally accepted scientific standards and should not cause harm. In 1979, the Belmont Report was published to guide the conducts of research. In 1981 and onwards, U.S. Federal Regulations at 45CFR Part 46 were promulgated and different guidelines issued by different organizations were published to focus on the ethical issue in different aspects (Grady, 2002). Regardless of codes or guidelines used in different counties and intuitions, the primary purpose of having ethical issues addressed in clinical research is to protect the subject while conducting a valid research. As Emanel, Wendler and Grady (2000) suggested, a systematic framework of principles that apply sequentially to all clinical research should be proposed based on the synthesis of guidance found. In the following part, we would discuss the requirements a clinical research hasve to fulfill in order to be ethical and the importance of satisfying the ethical principles.

Ethical Principles and its Importance

Although clinical research has produced substantial social benefits through generating practical knowledge to advance medical care and health,; it continues to pose some ethical dilemmas to the researcher. According to Marks-Maran (1994), this requires researchers to examine their value and feelings as well as to apply knowledge of ethics and ethical principles to research-related ethical situations when coping with ethical issues in research. As mentioned by the University of Minnesota Center for Bioethics (2003) "all researchers should be familiar with the basic ethical principles and have up-to-date knowledge about policies and procedures designed to ensure the safety of research subjects and to prevent sloppy or irresponsible research" (p. 6). According to different literatures, different frameworks of principles have been proposed, some stated the basic ethical principles according to the principles in the Belmont report about respect for persons, beneficence and justice (Lo, Feigal, Cummins & Hulley, 1988; Derenzo & Moss, 2006; Chatburn, 2011); others modified theirs from the Belmont report with the non-maleficence added (French, Reynolds, & Swain, 2001); some used seven to eight principles that consist of namely, the valuable scientific question, valid scientific methodology, fair subject selection, favorable risk- benefit ratio, independent review, informed consent, respect for the enrolled subjects and with or without collaborative partnership (Grady, 2007; Emanel, Wendler & Grady, 2000); some even used more than eight ethical principles which included authorship, plagiarism, peer review, conflicts of interest, data management, misconduct in addition to the principles for research with human subjects (University of Minnesota Center for Bioethics, 2003). Although different taxonomies for identifying ethical principles have been used, they all aim at helping the researcher to achieve an ethical research. In this paper, ethical principles are divided into ethical principles for research with human subjectss and ethical principles concerning with the designation, conduction and publication of research. Different principles would be briefly elaborated and the importance of having the principles would be discussed.

I.   Respect for persons

The principle of respect for persons requires "respect for each individual's values, perspectives and capacities; assisting individuals in exercising self-determination; and the provision of appropriate protections for individuals who have limitations on autonomous behavior" (Derenzo & Moss, 2006, p.18). It is necessary for the researcher to obtain informed consent from participants to prevent deceit and coercion (Lo, 2007; Aveyard & Hawley, 2007). The participants enter into the research voluntarily with adequate information and can withdraw during the research process (Chatburn, 2011). Treating Pparticipants as partners helps increaseing their enrollment and compliance, thus, improving the scientific quality of the research (Lo, Feigal, Cummins & Hulley, 1988).

II.   Favorable risk-benefit ratio (Beneficence & non-maleficence)

The favorable risk-benefit ratio is positive when the benefits outweigh the risks (Grady, 2007). Beneficence and non-maleficence refer to bringing benefit to and not intentional or unintentional harm to research participants, respectively (Aveyard & Hawley, 2007; French, Reynolds & Swain, 2001). "It is a widely accepted principle that one should not deliberately harm another individual regardless of the benefits that might be made available to others" (Grady, 2007, p.21). The procedures to ensure a favorable risk-benefit ratio should be done before inviting an individual to a research, which is to guarantee the research being done in an ethical manner that is credible.

III. Justice (Fair subject selection)

The principle of justice refers to "being fair" (Holzemer, 2003, p.12). The benefits and burdens of research are required to be distributed fairly (Lo, 2007). Fair subject selection means the researcher has to select subjects based on the scientific question. This procedure should be balanced by considering the risk, benefit and vulnerability instead of focusing on the availability or manipulability (Emanel, Wendler, & Grady, 2000; Weijer, 2002). This is to prevent exploitation of stigmatized and vulnerable individuals for risky research and the rich and socially powerful being favored for potentially beneficial research (Emanel, Wendler, & Grady, 2000). Also, this is important for promoting equitable distribution of research burden and benefits as well as minimizing risk and maximizing benefit (Grady, 2007).

The involvement of humans in clinical research is ultimately important as no research can be done without human participation. The broadest objective of the above three ethical issues is to protect human participants by "minimizinge the possibility of exploitation by ensuring that research subjects are not merely used but are treated with respect while they contribute to the social good" (Emanel, Wendler & Grady, 2000, p.2701) and protecting their rights and welfare. This also ensures the results of the research arebeing credible. However, other than the ethical principles focused on research with human subjects, there are also some extra ethical principles that we have to address properly when designing, conducting and reporting the research to ensure our research integrity. By considering ethical issues from the conceptual stage of a proposal, the quality of research is enhanced.

IV.   Valuable scientific question & Valid scientific methodology

As stated by Grady (2007), ethical clinical research should answer a valuable question that might offer practical or useful knowledge to understand or improve health. This means the crucial criteria of a valuable scientific question is its usefulness in the knowledge gained. Also, ethical clinical research should be designed in a methodologically rigorous manner that is feasible, yielding valid, reliable, generalizable, and interpretable data (Grady, 2007). Value is required because it is unethical to expend resources or to ask individuals to assume risks or inconvenience for no socially valuable purpose (Freedman, 1987). Also validity is required as the research would cause a waste in human and material resources and expose participants to risk for no benefits if the research design is not valid, reliable and generalizable results cannot be produced (Emanel, Wendler, & Grady, 2000).

V.   Data management

According to the University of Minnesota Center for Bioethics (2003), data management refer to three issues: "the ethical and truthful collection of reliable data; the ownership and responsibility of collected data; and retaining data and sharing access to collected data with colleagues and the public" (p.22). In this instance, an ethical and truthful data collection includes assigning and ensuring responsibility for collecting and maintaining data helps to protect participants from harm; to ensure the data is not manipulated whichthat might results inof false findings; and to preserve the integrity and privacy of data (University of Minnesota Center for Bioethics, 2003). Data sharing is also one of the most important ethical considerations when conducting a research, although it helps encourage accuracy and verification of data, data associated with intellectual property needsed to be retained. It is important for the researcher to protect the intellectual property while at the same time encourage data sharing in order to ensure valid and reliable research (University of Minnesota Center for Bioethics, 2003).

VI.   Conflicts of interest

Conflicts of interest arise when a person (or an organization) involved in a particular research project conflict with their personal interests or obligations (National Institutes of Health, 2010). In clinical research, health care professional researchers may encounter conflicts of interest between their duties towards research and their duties towards the health and welfare of their patients (University of Minnesota Center for Bioethics, 2003). It is important to address conflicts of interest properly to promote objectivity in research and ensure unbiased design, conduct and reporting of the results (U.S Department of Health & Human Services, 2010). Without addressing conflicts of interest properly, the researchers are in great risk of losing support and respect from the public and lead to doom in clinical research (DeAngelis, 2000). Also, and particular to clinical research, obligations to patients should always be considered above and beyond the obligations of research for upholding the highest standards for patient safety.

VII.   Plagiarism

Plagiarism is using others' ideas or words without properly acknowledging the source of that information (The Hong Kong Polytechnic University, 2005). It is crucial in all means as it is viewed as an illegal act and considered stealing others' properties. In addition to ensuring the originality of work by punishing those plagiarists, in the research field, avoiding plagiarism helps to increase the chance of research manuscripts to be accepted by the publisher as plagiarism, which is non-tolerable, brings the integrity, ethics, and trustworthiness of the research into question and leads to the rejection of the research manuscripts by publishers (University of Minnesota Center for Bioethics, 2003).

VIII.   Authorship

Authorship refers to "the process of deciding whose names belong on a research paper" (University of Minnesota Center for Bioethics, 2003, p.8). It is important to have a proper authorship practices because it can protect the authors' work and ideas, as well as helping preventing research fraud by urging the author to take responsibilities of the study.

IX.   Collaborative partnership

Since research often involves a great deal of cooperation and coordination among many different people in different disciplines or institutions, ethical clinical research should be done in a collaborative partnership in order to conduct a good research (Resnik, 2010). Collaborative partnership also can be applied to the researcher and the participants in research; according to Lo, Feigal, Cummins and Hulley (1988), this helps to improve the scientific quality of the research by increasing enrollment and compliance. Thus, ethical principles which promote the values that are essential to collaborative work should be addressed sincerely.

All in all, ethical issues should be addressed properly since, in addition to protecting the subjects from potentially harmful practices (McNally, 2002), it also promotes the aims of the research while avoiding errors. It also provides moral and social values that are essential to collaborative work like responsibility (Resnik, 2010) and helps to protect the researcher from possible future legal difficulties (McNally, 2002). The ethical research can also be accountable to the public, thus, helps to build public support for the research (Resnik, 2010).

Conclusion

In conclusion, it is of fundamentally importancet for us to engage ethical issues in research properly and sincerely in order to provide valuable research. Throughout the history of research, there are unethical researches conducted, the accounting of these researches can provide important lessons for us to understand what can happen when ethical issues in research aredo not considered holistically. Nowadays, different ethical regulations or guidelines haves been permanently added in designing, conducting and evaluating the research. Although ethical issues are never the same in each clinical research, by understanding the ethical principles and the importance behind them, we will know how we should act and how we can solve the dilemma. It is the responsibility of the researcher to ensure that the principles of autonomy, beneficence, and justice are preserved as well as to cultivate a culture of research integrity when conducting a clinical research. Thus, ethical standards which serve as leading guidelines for correct research practice involving human participants must be understood and followed.

Author's Background

Lung Kwan Yu, Maggie, a year two student who is studying Master of Nursing in the Hong Kong Polytechnic University and the Hong Kong Sanatorium Hospital. (Email: makilung@gmail.com)

References

Aveyard, H., & Hawley, G. (2007). How to do ethical health care research. In G. Hawley (Ed.), *Ethics in clinical practice: An interprofessional approach* (pp. 348-365). Harlow, England: Pearson Education.

Chatburn, R. L. (2011). *Handbook for health care research* (2nd ed.). Sudbury, Mass.: Jones and Bartlett publisher.

Council for International Organizations of Medical Sciences, & World Health Organization. (2002). *International ethical guidelines for biomedical research involving human subjects*. Retrieved October 27, 2010, from http://whqlibdoc.who.int/emro/2004/9290213639_annex2.pdf

DeAngelis, C. D. (2000). Conflicts of interest and the public trust. *Journal of the American Medical Association, 284*(17), 2237-2238.

Derenzo, E., & Moss, J. (2006). *Writing clinical research protocols: Ethical considerations*. London: Elsevier Academic Press.

Emanel, E., Wendler, D., & Grady, C. (2000). What makes clinical research ethical? *Journal of the American Medical Association, 283*(20), 2701-2711.

Freedman, B. (1987). Scientific value and validity as ethical requirements for research: A proposed explanation. *Review Human Subjects Research, 9*(5), 7-10.

French, S., Reynolds, F., & Swain, J. (2001). *Practical research: A guide for therapists* (2nd ed.). Oxford: Butterworth-Heinemann.

Grady, C. (2002). Ethical principles in clinical research. In J. I. Gallin (Eds.), *Principles and practice of clinical research* (pp.15-26).New York: Academic Press.

Grady, C. (2007). Ethical principles in clinical research. In J. I. Gallin, & F. P. Ognibene (Eds.), *Principles and practice of clinical research* (2nd ed., pp.15-26). New York: Elsevier, Academic Press.

Hesse-Biber, S. N., & Leavy, P. (2006). *The practice of qualitative research.* Los Angeles: Sage.

Holzemer, W. L. (2003). *Ethical guidelines for nursing research.* Geneva: International Council of Nurses.

Jones, J. H. (1993). *Bad Blood: The Tuskegee experiment.* New York: Free Press.

Lo, B. (2007). Addressing Ethical Issues. In S. B. Hulley, S.R. Cummings, W. S. Browner, D. G. Grady, & T.B. Newman (Eds.), *Designing clinical research* (3rd ed., pp. 225-240). Philadelphia, PA: Lippincott William & Wilkins.

Lo, B., Feigal, D., Cummins, S., & Hulley, S. B. (1988). Addressing ethical issue. In S. B. Hulley, & S. R. Cummins (Eds.), *Designing clinical research: An epidemiologic approach* (pp.151-158). Baltimore: Williams & Wilkins.

Marks-Maran, D. (1994). Nursing research. In V. Tschudin (Ed.), *Ethics: Education and research* (pp.40-71). London: Scutari Press.

McNally, P. (2002). How to get started in clinical research. In J.Niebauer (Ed.) *The clinical research survival guide* (pp.21-41). London: Remedica.

National Institutes of Health. (2010). *Conflict of Interest.* Retrieved November 7, 2010, from http://ethics.od.nih.gov/topics/coi.htm

Resnik, D. R. (2010). *What is ethics in research & why is it important?* Retrieved October 27, 2010, from http://www.niehs.nih.gov/research/resources/bioethics/whatis.cfm

Talbot, D., & Perou, J. (2001). Ethical issues. In I. D. Giovanna, & G. Hayes (Eds.), *Principles of clinical research* (pp.63-83). Petersfield: Wrightson Biomedical.

The Hong Kong Polytechnic University. (2005). *Being professional in your studies.* Retrieved November 3, 2010, from http://edc.polyu.edu.hk/PSP/student.htm

UNAIDS. (2007). *Ethical considerations in biomedical HIV prevention trial.* Retrieved November 1, 2010, from http://data.unaids.org/pub/Report/2007/JC1399_ethical_considerations_en.pdf

University of Minnesota Center for Bioethics. (2003). *A guide to research ethics.* Retrieved November 1, 2010, from http://www.ahc.umn.edu/img/assets/26104/Research_Ethics.pdf

U.S Department of Health & Human Services. (2010). *Financial conflict of interest.* Retrieved November 7, 2010, from http://grants.nih.gov/grants/policy/coi/

Weijer, C. (2002). Ethics in clinical research. In J. Niebauer (Ed.), *The clinical research survival guide* (pp.79-92). London: Remedica.

World Medical Association. (2008). *WMA Declaration of Helsinki: Ethical Principles for Medical Research Involving Human Subjects.* Retrieved November 1, 2010, from http://www.wma.net/en/30publications/10policies/b3/index.html

Index

disclosure, 173
discrete data, 98
discrimination, 123, 125
diseases, 58
dispersion, 105
distress, 92
distribution, 84, 90, 96, 97, 99, 100, 188
diversification, 5
diversity, 164, 166
doctors, 4, 122
DOI, 85, 86
drawing, 59, 75, 104
drinking water, 158
drug abuse, 48
drugs, 48
dualism, 26

E

education, vii, 1, 2, 3, 4, 5, 6, 8, 15, 60, 63, 80, 99,
    151, 155, 160, 163, 165
educational programs, 74
educational research, 167
educators, 27
e-learning, 40
elementary school, 165
elementary students, 165
eligibility criteria, 84
elucidation, 106
emboli, 59
empathy, 150, 174
empirical methods, 162
energy, 2, 58, 142
England, 49, 101, 109, 151, 191
enrollment, 188, 190
environment, 2, 38, 44, 46, 59, 65, 178, 179, 180,
    182
environmental factors, 178
environmental impact, 1
epidemiology, 57, 60
epistemology, vii, viii, 7, 10, 15, 17, 33, 34, 40
equal opportunity, 163
equality, 3
equilibrium, 164
equipment, 89
ethical issues, x, xii, 87, 92, 166, 178, 185, 186, 187,
    189, 190, 191
ethical standards, 191
ethics, 175, 179, 186, 187, 190, 192
ethnic groups, 156
ethnographers, 156
everyday life, 68, 154

evidence, vii, viii, xii, 1, 2, 4, 15, 19, 20, 49, 57, 59,
    60, 70, 76, 77, 101, 111, 116, 120, 124, 129,
    142, 143, 146, 167, 169, 170, 175, 178, 180,
    183, 185
evolution, 14
exclusion, 70, 80, 84
exercise, 174
experimental design, 10, 20, 48, 49, 54, 56, 57, 99,
    126, 167, 178, 179
expertise, 173
exploitation, 188, 189
exposure, 108
external validity, 83, 115, 120, 125, 170
extraction, 91
extraneous variable, 70, 123, 124, 125, 178, 180

F

face validity, 112, 122
facilitators, 181, 184
factor analysis, 114
factual knowledge, 16
faith, 35
families, 119, 152, 156, 182, 183
family income, 47
family members, 3, 41, 180, 181
family system, 3
fantasy, 59
fear, 130
feelings, xi, 19, 36, 91, 123, 150, 153, 187
flaws, 44
flexibility, 26
fluctuations, 140
focus groups, xi, 48, 62, 161, 163, 181
formula, 82, 137, 139
foundations, 15, 77
fraud, 190
freedom, 28
frequency distribution, 104, 105
fruits, 57
funding, 84, 147

G

general knowledge, 155, 156
generalizability, ix, xi, 19, 39, 69, 74, 79, 80, 82, 84,
    126, 159, 161, 162, 163, 164, 165, 166, 167,
    182
glasses, 135
graduate program, 3
grants, 192
grass, 181